TIME FOR A
HEART-TO-HEART

ALSO BY BOB MITCHELL

Everything on the Line (novel)

Once Upon a Fastball (novel)

Match Made in Heaven (novel)

*How My Mother Accidentally Tossed Out
My Entire Baseball-Card Collection*
(essays)

The Tao of Sports (prose poems)

The Heart Has Its Reasons (poems)

TIME FOR A HEART-TO-HEART

Reflections on Life in the Face of Death

Bob Mitchell

FOREWORD BY LARRY KING

Skyhorse Publishing

Skyhorse Publishing books may be purchased in bulk at special discounts for sales promotion, corporate gifts, fund-raising, or educational purposes. Special editions can also be created to specifications. For details, contact the Special Sales Department, Skyhorse Publishing, 307 West 36th Street, 11th Floor, New York, NY 10018 or info@skyhorsepublishing.com.

Skyhorse® and Skyhorse Publishing® are registered trademarks of Skyhorse Publishing, Inc.®, a Delaware corporation.

Visit our website at www.skyhorsepublishing.com.
Visit Bob Mitchell's website at www.bobmitchellheart2heart.com.

10 9 8 7 6 5 4 3 2 1

Library of Congress Cataloging-in-Publication Data is available on file.

Cover design by Rain Saukas
Author photograph by Susan Ellen Love

Print ISBN: 978-1-5107-2440-2
Ebook ISBN: 978-1-5107-2441-9

Printed in the United States of America.

Again, to Susan Ellen Love, from the bottom of my heart.

Midway through our life's journey
I found myself in a dark wood.
—Dante Alighieri

Don't it always seem to go
That you don't know what you've got till it's gone?
—Joni Mitchell

A Wounded *Deer—leaps highest—*
—Emily Dickinson

Do not go gentle into that good night.
Rage, rage against the dying of the light.
—Dylan Thomas

The heart has its reasons that reason doesn't have a clue about.
—Blaise Pascal

I ain't never saw a hearse with a luggage rack.
—George Strait

Contents

Foreword

A decade ago, Bob Mitchell asked me to write a blurb for the cover of his baseball novel, *Once Upon a Fastball*, which I gladly did. I liked his writing, and, besides, although I didn't know him personally, I figured we Brooklyn-born-and-bred sports fanatics with serious heart issues have to stick together, right? And now, I'm pleased to be writing the foreword to this unusual memoir about his recent cardiac saga and survival.

When it comes to affairs of the heart, well, I've been around the block a few times. In 1987, when I had my quintuple-bypass surgery, heart disease suddenly became a big part of my life, and ever since, I've tried my best to help others who struggle with it.

Likewise, Bob Mitchell's memoir—a thoughtful and pro-vocative account of his life-threatening heart disease and trans-plant surgery, and of his one-hundred-day physical and mental ordeal in various hospitals—will certainly help others, and their families and friends, who find themselves in a similar situation.

There are lots of memoirs out there about heart disease, but *Time for a Heart-to-Heart* is unique. It's not just a narra-tive of someone enduring the obvious pain and anxiety that accompany a prolonged hospital stay culminating (at last!) in a heart transplant. On a deeper level, it tackles many of the serious conflicts in life that Bob pondered during his ordeal and about which he has been thinking, teaching, and writing for more than five decades: fear and hope, humility and pride, and control and surrender, to name a few. There are important lessons to be learned here, for sure.

Bob's memoir has a lot going for it. On the one hand, it's a poignant piece of writing, coming straight from his cardiac muscle. He expresses his inner thoughts and memories in a powerful, moving way that humanizes the whole experience of what it's like to be at death's doorstep and waiting for a new organ. On the other hand, it's thought-provoking and challenging, with lots of insight and wisdom, inviting any reader with a beating heart to contemplate nothing less than the meaning of life. Plus, it's a fun read filled with entertaining anecdotes from Bob's colorful past. As we used to say in Brooklyn, "What's not to like?"

I know that if I say this is a "must read," it might come off as sounding a little cliché. But, hey, I can't help myself. This is a must read.

Enjoy!

Larry King
Founder, Larry King Cardiac Foundation
April 2016

TIME FOR A
HEART-TO-HEART

1
Do-Over

Eyewitnesses have testified under oath that on the morning of November 6, 1944, I exited my mother's birth canal sporting a teeny pair of Rawlings baseball spikes. A tad painful for my mom, they recall, but a scenario not too far-fetched now to those who know me well.

Soon thereafter, my little feet grew by proverbial leaps and bounds and during the next seventeen years gleefully inhabited, in turn, Converse tennis sneakers, Chuck Taylor basketball sneakers, Adidas soccer cleats, and FootJoy golf shoes. And ever since, sports has been an integral part of my life.

My formative years—spent in Brooklyn, NY—were largely dominated by and filled themselves constantly, passionately, with nothing more complicated than the febrile joy of athletic competition. From my prepubescent days to my midteens, I spent seemingly endless hours flipping baseball cards ("heads and tails," "leaners"); creating and playing in melodramatic and imaginary contests with my trusty "Spaldeen" rubber ball, including the madcap "Bottom of the Ninth," in which my beloved NY Giants would invariably stage a miraculous rally against the Bums or Phils or Cards in their last licks to pull the game out of their collective cloacal orifice; playing concocted maniacal games like basement hockey and hangerball, which featured a bent wire hanger masquerading as a basketball hoop wedged between frame and closed bedroom door and a pair of rolled-up white Wigwam socks that I "air-dribbled" against an imaginary defender; and competing in frog races against my older brother (in the fifties, these speckled beauts—*rana pipiens*—were used by pathologists for pregnancy tests: don't even ask . . .) on the floor of my father's medical lab, which I affectionately christened "the Pipidrome."

It is early November, 1953, in Brooklyn, and I have just turned nine. I am a high-metabolism, high-energy, low-patience fourth-grader. I am the great-grandfather of the Energizer Bunny. My heart is strong, my body is strong, I am a whirling dervish except when I am asleep (and even then, my dreams are probably racing at 78 rpm). My middle name is Trouble. My mom calls me a *vontz* (mischief-maker, literally Yiddish for "bedbug"). I call myself Bobby.

Many of my memories of Brooklyn in those olden days are somewhat faded now, but certain recollections of my neighborhood—the Borough Park section—remain ridiculously fresh in my mind. I can still smell the bananas from the peddlers' rickety green carts, the sour pickles and kippered herrings from Miller's Appetizer, the pastrami and knishes from Skilowitz and Hoffinger's delicatessens, the blackout cakes and huckleberry crumb pies from Ebinger's bakery, the egg creams and malteds from Hessing's corner luncheonette. I can still see the storefronts from yesterdecade that have long ago disappeared: Linick's Toys (I used to purchase my Spaldeens and Red Ryder comic books there), Jaynel's Records (where I bought my first phonograph record in 1956, a 78 rpm of Elvis, with "Don't Be Cruel" on the "A" side and "Hound Dog" on the "B"), Moe Penn Haberdashers (most men wore actual hats back then!), Rothstein's Clothing, El-Gee Electric, the Manny Hanny Bank, The Famous vegetarian restaurant, Al del Gaudio's barber shop, G & Sons department store, Woolworth's five-and-dime, and Monty Greenhut's Mobil station, with its polite cap- and uniform-bedecked attendants. I can still envision the curbs on each side of the streets bloated—fat bumper-to-fat bumper— with obese, lumpy cars, long-forgotten brands like DeSotos, Hudsons, Packards, Nashes, Henry Js, and Studebakers. I can still feel in my bones the intensity and mutual hatred of the Dodgers-Giants baseball rivalry (the Dodgers purportedly hated Halloween because its colors—orange and black—were also those of the detested Giants). Contrarian that I was, and still am, I was one of the very few rabid Giants fans to be found anywhere in the borough.

Way back in those Jurassic days, life was pretty simple. The US wasn't at war, the Korean conflict having ended the previous July. Electronic devices were limited to boxy, behemoth black telephones with rotary dials and six-foot, inevitably tangled curly handset cords; twelve-inch-screen TVs in mahogany frames with clunky little wheels you turned around and around to reach the seven (you heard me, *seven*) available stations; and tubby radios with netted openings, dials galore, and a red needle you moved painstakingly with a knob to indicate the next station (that is, if you could ever locate it). If you wanted to open a can or a garage door or squeeze fresh OJ, well, you had to do it manually. No remote or automatic anythings for anything. Many eons before computers and smartphones, if you needed to write something down, you used a scrap of paper and a good ol' #2 Eberhard Faber Mongol lead pencil. And the *New York Times* cost just an Indian Head nickel.

Choosing loyalties was a pretty simple proposition, too. A real no-brainer, in fact, because there seemed to be only two viable choices for each category. Fab or Tide? Colgate or Ipana? Ford or Chevy? Magnavox or Philco? Corn Flakes or Rice Krispies? Roy Rogers or Gene Autry? Oh Henry! or Hershey's? Corned beef or pastrami? Betty or Veronica?

Similarly, back then, active, red-blooded nine-year-olds in Brooklyn didn't have too many options for things to keep them busy. Nope, I sure didn't sit around playing video games or texting friends or Googling or tweeting. In fact, all I really needed to survive—aside from eating three squares a day and snacking all day long and attending public school—was my trusty Spaldeen (Brooklynese pronunciation: SPAWL-DEEN), a local way to say the brand name "Spalding." Grab my Spaldeen in my grimy little palm, and I was good to go. To keep myself busy and happy, I'd play with it in my driveway for three, four hours a day, between end of school and beginning of dinner. It was my best, and most trusted, friend in life.

The Spaldeen was a pink rubber honey of a ball you could squish with your knuckles to make it curve or even come back to you after bouncing forward. It was firm yet pliable; and, as a bonus, it exuded the pristine odor of talcumy powder when you bought it, an aroma that fostered feelings of well-being and desire. Then, there were no iPhones or smartphones to waste your time with. Only Spaldeens.

And, ah, the games I played! Stoopball, brickball, boxball, wallball, curbball, angleball, garage-doorball, anything my little hyperkinetic mind could concoct that required skill and creativity, and that stoked my white-hot competitive fires.

So, one Tuesday morning in November of 1953, during recess, I am standing on the sidewalk just outside the playground of my elementary school, P. S. 180, on Fifty-Sixth Street and Sixteenth Avenue. Facing me is Michael Krumholz, my best pal and fellow mischief-maker. We are engaged in a hot-and-heavy, fiercely competitive game of pennyball.

Because of its purity and simplicity, pennyball is the ultimate Zen sport. All you need is a penny, a Spaldeen, and a sidewalk with cracks. That's it.

Here's how it works. You and your opponent choose any three consecutive cracks in a sidewalk. You station yourself behind one of the outer cracks, your opponent stations himself behind the other outer crack, and the penny is placed smack in the middle of the center crack. Then, you take turns tossing the Spaldeen overhand—the short takeback, wrist snap, and abbreviated follow-through resemble those employed in a game of darts—at the penny (which moves, of course, either toward you or away from you after impact), and you get one point every time you hit it. The first to reach an agreed-upon point total (usually ten or twenty-five) wins.

Despite appearing ostensibly unathletic and boring, penny-ball is actually an extremely demanding game, requiring skill, discipline, focus, self-control, resilience, finesse, endurance, hand-eye coordination, and poise. And if anyone who lacks the knowledge of Brooklynese history and culture should dare say otherwise, you can just tell them two things, and you can say you heard them from me: *You're so funny, I forgot to laugh* and *Up your nose with a rubber hose.*

Anyway, there we are, Michael Krumholz and I, standing on the sidewalk and facing each other, red-faced from the intensity of the battle, our visages twisted in maniacal poses, our lips clenched from the insane preadolescent desire to vanquish and humiliate our opponent.

It is Michael's turn, and he's between a coin and a hard place. It is 24-23, favor of me, and he needs to hit the penny to tie the game and preserve his slim chances of winning. (Even if he gets a point now, I win, 25-24, if I score when it's my turn.)

"Feeling the pressure, eh?" I taunt. Michael shoots me a quick Dick Cheney snarl, unwilling to dignify my snide remark with a rejoinder.

I can feel his little mind being squished in the vice of tension. I can see the beads of sweat forming on his troubled brow. I can almost taste the sweet wine of Victory.

The penny he is aiming at is in his box, only two feet or so from where he is positioned, so the degree of difficulty of his chances of hitting it is about a two on a scale of one to ten, unbearable pressure notwithstanding.

Imaginary drum roll. Michael's eyes, focusing intently on his target, metamorphose into tiny slits. A pregnant pause of four seconds, then, at the exact instant that the end-of-recess alarm sounds, the Spaldeen leaves his hand and wends its way toward the penny. And, by no more than a hundredth of a speck . . . *it misses!*

"Yay!" I shout, with unabashedly explosive joy.

Michael is crushed, but, unsurprisingly, he refuses to admit defeat.

"*Hey!*" he whines, "the game's not over. I get another chance. You heard that alarm bell, didn't you? I got distracted, couldn't concentrate. *I deserve another chance!*"

"No do-overs!" I screech adamantly. "You had your turn, fair and square, and I won!"

"*Did not!*" Krumholz snivels.

"*Did too!*" I retort maturely. "Listen, you sore loser, didn't you ever hear of integrity? My dad taught me all about it, and how you have to do what's right, even if it hurts you."

Michael's mouth opens wide, an uncomprehending look fills his startled face.

"In other words, *no do-overs!*" I repeat even more frantically, my face turning beet. "No second chances! You get one shot. That's the whole point!" I am passionate (and admittedly self-righteous) about this, about the fact that do-overs—in penny-ball as in life—are simply not acceptable and in fact must be avoided on pain of death.

It will be a mere sixty-two years later that I realize how very mistaken I was.

2
Dark Wood

Lying prone on my seventy-year-old belly, here I am, in April of 2015, a lifelong sports fanatic and former semipro soccer player and teaching tennis pro, attempting to slither my way ever-so-painstakingly—at the approximate rate of one every twenty-four seconds—up the fourteen steps leading to my writing study in Carlsbad, CA.

My heart is very sick. Ever since I had several coronary infarctions and quadruple-bypass surgery in 1986, it has eventually lost muscle to the point of now being comprised of 54 percent scar tissue. After a few more heart attacks and angioplasties and stents, it has only one functioning major coronary artery left now, and the great irony is that it is my circumflex artery and I was a French professor for many years (the circumflex is an accent mark in French). Further, because of my heart's screwed-up "electrical system," I had a defibrillator inserted in my chest in 1998, to correct the various arrhythmias I had accrued, like atrial fibrillation and—even more foreboding—the potentially fatal ventricular tachydardia. Because these abnormal heartbeats have worsened so much and so steadily, my heart's days as a viable pump are now officially numbered. So much so that I can barely climb stairs or walk ten steps or even tie my shoes without experiencing shortness of breath and of optimism.

Gasping for air, I pause, and my idiosyncratic mind naturally meanders to the opening verses of thirty-five-year-old Dante's fourteenth-century masterpiece, *Inferno*:

> *Midway through our life's journey*
> *I found myself in a dark wood.*

In my snail-like stupor, I realize that the life span in Dante's time was seventy. *Seventy!* And now, at the very age of seventy, I find myself in my own *selva oscura*, my own "dark wood," this terrifying forest of confusion and fear, the darkest, in fact, of all the dark woods of my life.

I am thinking of how intriguing it is that Dante used the expression "*our* life" instead of "*my* life," and the universality of it: we all experience this "wood" of confusion and fear at some point—the death of family members or friends; money, work, or relationship problems; serious health issues; whatever. And it is occurring to me that I am not here just struggling alone pathetically, but that I am also part of nothing less than the human condition.

Yet it sure feels lonely now. I am in my little cocoon of pain and helplessness, and, to boot, my beloved wife, Susan, just so happens to be at the gym working out.

Crawling up one more step, I realize all too clearly that I am in deep shit. Well, let me qualify that. In 1985, when I was an advertising copywriter, I partnered with an incredibly talented art director from Durban, South Africa, named Seymon Ostilly. Once, stumped by a particular project and temporarily unable to come up with any intelligent solutions for an ad concept (as often happened), I announce to him, "Seymon, we're in profound caca!" He laughs and says, "Hang on a bit," and then, his eyes emitting a creative glimmer, he draws a hasty but artful little cartoon of a massively thick and tall pyramid-shaped mound of fecal matter with two stick figures trapped in the middle of it, scribbles PROFOUND CACA as the caption at the bottom, and attaches it with two brightly colored push pins onto the back of the door. Instantly, it becomes a constant reminder to us of the difficulty of art (and of life) and the need to inject humor into our most challenged moments.

But now, in profound caca, I find nothing remotely funny about my present challenged moment. In fact, I am feeling pretty much like a failure, which is not like me at all. To cheer myself up, I summon a quote from a Chinese book of wisdom written over 2,500 years ago, Lao-tzu's *Tao Te Ching*: "Failure is an opportunity." And consider how, in my life, losing has taught me a great deal more than winning has.

While I was in high school, for instance, I won over fifty tennis singles matches and lost three. To this day, I have no recollection of anyone I ever beat. But I can recite the specifics of the losses—names of opponents, scores, and, most important, the lessons I learned and what I did to improve and elevate my game thereafter. This ability to learn and improve after a loss is a sort of self-repechage, a gift you can give yourself in order to get better.

And when I lost my job in advertising in the early 1990s, I learned—once again—all about shock and disappointment and panic. And how to deal with these issues and bounce back and believe more than ever in myself and move on.

So this begs the (particularly all-American) question: Why is *not losing* so important to us? Sports (and life, for that matter) is a game of inches, so what's the big freaking deal? Why are we so obsessed with success and winning, when their existence is so fragile, so short-lived, so dependent on so little? An inch here or there, and the result is different. Not only does losing not reflect a shortcoming or character flaw in us, but the benefits it offers (life lessons, learning, improvement, character building) far outweigh its liabilities.

But back to Lao-tzu's quote: What opportunity, what lessons, what silver lining can *this* miserable failure lead to? What can I learn from my present nightmare? In this moment, crawling up the stairs like an arthritic sloth, I'm stumped. I'm usually able to come up with an answer to such rhetorical questions, but now, frankly, I ain't in no mood.

I have reached the landing now, step #7, and I'm looking up at the 4' x 4' assemblage of my entire life that Susan (a wonderfully talented artist) lovingly and masterfully constructed for me in 2001, a few months after we first met and fell in love. Hung on the wall at the landing, it is a huge, multilayered, multileveled arrangement of the highlights of my life until the beginning of the new millennium, all displayed under a thick plexiglass cover.

These highlights include old photos, artifacts, caps, a tennis racquet and ball, a soccer jersey, a golf ball, membership cards,

books I had written, and various memorabilia, divided loosely
into sections, each one of which is now evoking in me, mercifully, all kinds of warm feelings and desperately needed distractions and still-vivid memories:

France. A *Taride* metro map of Paris, maps of the fifth and
sixth arrondissements, my old Parisian *Bibliothèque Nationale*
(National Library) card, my *Carte Orange* (public transportation
card), an article in the regional newspaper *Le Courrier de l'Ouest*
reviewing a folk concert performed by me and two other American musicians (Chuck Perrin, Lance Davis) at the Salle St.-
Laud in Nantes in 1967, old photos of Le Mont-Saint-Michel
in Normandy and of me standing in front of the poet Apolli-
naire's tomb in the Père Lachaise cemetery in Paris, the covers
of four books on French poetry that I wrote in the seventies, a
photo of me rollerblading in the Parisian suburb of Issy-les-
Moulineaux, a poster of a lecture I gave in 1977 on the poet
Tristan Corbière at the Weston Language Center at Williams
College, my alma mater.

Academia. Williams: my varsity soccer jersey, photos of me
and my then-girlfriend Dominique and of my two French men-
tors (Jack Savacool and George Pistorius), my Phi Beta Kappa
key, photos of me and the varsity soccer team and of me drib-
bling past a Bowdoin College defender, a photo of me giving
a spontaneous (and inebriated) twenty-minute lecture on the
History of Art from the Caveman to the Present at Professor
Fred Rudolph and wife Dottie's house in June of 1966 just after
graduation; Harvard: a University Officer's Card and a university seal; Ohio State: a Faculty Club card and a cardboard
ticket stub from an Ohio State-Michigan football game.

NY Giants. A black cap with orange (intertwined "NY") lettering, baseball cards of Willie Mays and Sal Maglie, an old black-and-white photo of Willie making that famous catch off Indians slugger Vic Wertz in the first game of the 1954 World Series, a photo of Bobby Thomson hitting that classic and iconic home run off Ralph Branca in the third and deciding game of the 1951 National League Pennant series, a miniature image of a felt black-and-orange Giants pennant featuring the Polo Grounds and Willard Mullin's cartoon of the childlike New York Giant.

Diving. My PADI Advanced Open Water Diver card, photos in Maui of me and skipper Pierre on his dive boat and of me and former girlfriend Diane sixty feet below the surface of the Pacific, a Maui Dive Shop decal.

Tennis. A cap from the Israeli Tennis Center in Ramat Hasharon, photos of me hitting with pal Mike Appelbaum in Florida and of me and John Newcombe at his Texas tennis ranch, my Northern California USTA 5.0 rating card, a tattered and faded green paper ticket from the 1959 Lawn Tennis Championships (Wimbledon) finals where Alex Olmedo beat an up-and-coming Rod Laver in straight sets, my (very) old Dunlop Maxpli wooden racquet, a Tretorn X tennis ball I used while giving lessons many decades ago.

Golf. My Titleist 1 golf ball that helped win the father-and-son tournament at the Inwood Country Club in Long Island in 1960, a scorecard from Inwood when I first broke 80.

My youth. A Spaldeen (of course!), a photo from 1947 of me and my older brother in front of Cape Cod Candies in Hyannis, a snapshot from 1949 of me in front of Papa Moe's 1946

Oldsmobile at his and Grandma Elsie's house at 1515 Forty-Eighth Street in Brooklyn, a baby picture of me on my belly (a frightening harbinger of . . . *now?*), a photo of me and my dad at Owl's Head Park in Brooklyn, a photo of me hitting a softball at Camp Dellwood in Honesdale, PA, at the age of six.

My dogs. Photos (in chronological order) of Job, Maglie, Mocha, and Koslo.

Books. Copies of three of my books: *The Heart Has Its Reasons* (poems), *The Tao of Sports* (prose poems), and *How My Mother Accidentally Tossed Out My Entire Baseball-Card Collection* (essays).

People. Photos of Susan and me; of my kids, Noah, Jenny, and Sarah; and of me and dear friends Mark Cripps (along with a 2000 NatWest Trophy Final ticket stub at Lord's Cricket Ground in London), Frank Fleizach, Hank and Elayne Gardstein, Bob Joseph and Val Light, Mike Appelbaum, Hugh Herbert-Burns, Seymon Ostilly, Al Gorfin and Anthony Caprio, David Frantz and John Gabel, Leo and Margaret Schwartz (and their kids, Ruthie and Daniel), Kenny and Paula Horn, Bill and Beth Jaquith, Pierre Vagneux (and his folks, André and Andrée), Lance and Mary Donaldson-Evans, Rony and Rachel Herz, Diane Cabaud (and her girls, Nicole and Simone), Pete and Linda Haller.

I have passed this lovely work of art every day many times, and each time I do, I take a few seconds—maybe thirty-seven or so—to gaze at it, always appreciating both the artfulness and the finesse it required from Susan to construct it and the deeply personal meaning it has for me. It has become a sort of affirmation, a visible, almost palpable symbol of the fact that my life is and has been worth something and has not been meaningless, that I have lived life passionately, have from time to time achieved my goals, and have given and received some joy to and from others.

And now, on step #7, Susan's assemblage is compelling me to consider the trajectory of my life, all the ups and downs and close calls, the joys and disappointments, the many different stages and phases, childhood, education, four professions, living all over the world, my writing, my sports, my dogs, my family and friends, Susan . . . In short, I am feeling, viscerally, that cliched "life-flashing-before-my-eyes" thing. How much time has elapsed and how much has happened to me during my lifetime! And after all that, here I am now, reduced to crawling up these stairs on my belly. I am thinking now about the truth of that lovely, pithy couplet "The Span of Life" by the poet Robert Frost:

The old dog barks backwards without getting up.
I can remember when he was a pup.

I first read this as a much younger man and remember thinking that, without a doubt, I'd never feel like that old dog. Well, guess what.

And then, suddenly, it hits me.

Has it all come to this?

In the fog of my dark wood, I am flashing back to a scene at home in Brooklyn on October 3, 1951, with nearly-seven-year-old me in front of an ancient mahogany Dumont TV with its twelve-inch screen, watching Bobby (another Bobby!) Thomson hit that epic home run off Ralph Branca in the greatest, most dramatic moment in the history of sports (don't get me started . . .) to win the pennant for my cherished NY Giants.

I am pondering the impossibility of it all, the Giants being behind by a seemingly insurmountable 4-1 deficit in the bottom of the ninth, their last licks, with one out. *Is there any hope?* my dispirited voice queries. *No way they can come back,* I remember thinking before the thrilling crack of the bat and the absurdly impossible happens.

Hey, ya never know!

My mind's eye is now envisioning that famous *Chicago Daily Tribune* headline: Dewey Defeats Truman.

I am picturing many of the examples in sports of startling upsets I have witnessed ever since I was a kid, hey-ya-never-know moments seared into my gray matter that I will take to my grave, examples of the unforeseen that have always inspired me to hope against all odds: Jack Fleck shocking the world by beating Ben Hogan in a Sunday golf playoff at the 1955 US Open, Cassius Clay's stunning upset of Sonny Liston to become heavyweight boxing champion in 1964, the virtually unknown and all-black Texas Western Miners upsetting all-white Kentucky in the NCAA basketball finals of 1966, the Jets fulfilling Joe Namath's ridiculous prediction by whipping Johnny Unitas's heavily favored Colts in the 1969 Super Bowl, the upstart NY Mets overcoming the cinch-to-win, sure-bet Orioles in the World Series that same year, fifty-five-year-old former champion and con artist Bobby Riggs dispatching of world's #1 women's tennis player thirty-year-old Margaret Court in 1973, the US Olympic hockey team beating the unbeatable Russians in 1980, North Carolina State shocking the mighty Houston Cougars in the 1983 NCAA basketball finals . . .

Speaking of which, as Coach Jimmy Valvano said at the 1993 ESPYs as he was dying of cancer, "Don't give up . . . don't ever give up." And as the poet Alexander Pope said, "Hope springs eternal in the human breast." In times of stress, duress, and direness, hopelessness can become hope, which can save a life. Attitude can get us through, and never more so did I consider this than here on my belly on the stairs.

I have somehow scratched and clawed my way to the penultimate step now, #13. I am a fighter. I am *not* going to croak here, pathetic and alone, crawling up the stairs on my belly. There *is* hope for me, I *am* going to get through this, goddammit. If *that* Bobby could perform a miracle, *this* one surely can!

With not a little melancholy, I am remembering how very fit I used to be in bygone years. The grueling soccer practices in high school and college. The long and hard-fought tennis matches. The energy and grit demanded by my college squash regimen. But most of all, among all these past crucibles of struggle, the marathon hangerball games I played against high school chum and rival Jimmy Blumstein in his house on East Twenty-Fourth Street (between Avenues N and O) in Flatbush.

I am picturing us, one of us crazy lunatic kids wildly toting this rolled-up-sock-ball-thing in his sweaty little palm, bouncing up and down to the soundless rhythm of his fake-dribble, menacing his stealthy way toward a floating ersatz coat hanger-basket squeezed between frame and closed door, while the other is bumping, shoving, pushing him away from his intended destination with Chuck Bednarik-like fury, shadowing, all over him like a rash. All of this adolescent lunacy is transpiring in dogged, earnest silence, with only the grunts and muffled ouches of battle intruding themselves, as if apologetically, into the intense, excruciating noiselessness. And the prolific scoring would go on and on, despite the unyielding, grinding defense. And so would the groaning and the moaning and the sweating and the bruising and the pushing and the pulling and the bumping and the grinding. Until, after four hours or so, exhausted, spent, and collapsed in a massive heap on the floor in the middle of his bedroom, Jimmy and I would at last, begrudgingly, agree to call it quits at 662-662.

I have now reached the top step, the second-story floor, and I am sitting on my sorry ass, gazing into space. Gasping for air, I am mumbling to myself, in ascending agony, "Oh *boy*," then, "Oh *man*," then, "Oh *God*," exactly the same expressions I recall uttering during my very first myocardial infarction that I suffered in 1986, just before I took a ride in an ambulance to Montefiore Medical Center in the Bronx to have quadruple-bypass surgery. And I suddenly realize now, after lo these three decades, that these three utterances reflect—consciously or coincidentally?—a linguistic progression and a weirdly logical, albeit panicky, evolutionary escalation.

I finally reach my study. I can barely breathe now. I have not yet called Susan on her cell because I have yet to get to mine, which is on my writing desk. And now, I am too stupid to call because I am still, somehow, a cockeyed optimist and have some ludicrously moronic (male?) pride that is telling me I will recover very quickly and all will be well and she will come home soon anyway. I am by now in seriously profound caca and denial, and I desperately need to inject some humor into the situation. And *pronto*.

Sure enough, a funny incident (hilarious, in fact, to me at the time) floats into my brain that happens to be eerily appropriate for the occasion. I call it "The Torre Story."

The year is 2001, and my life is at a crossroads. I have just spent a year in Europe, trying to reenter advertising—my royalties for various published books have been dwindling, as has my pathetic bank account—as an international creative director at agencies mostly in Paris, but also in Stockholm, London, and Tel Aviv. It doesn't quite work out, so I have returned to the States and am spending a few weeks in Palm Beach Gardens, FL, with my parents. Deciding what to do with my life and where in the world to relocate. I have spent more than a week playing tennis with my old friend, fellow teaching tennis pro Mike Appelbaum, and golf with my dad and cogitating about my plans for the future and the meaning of life and making tons of lists and trying to make sense of it all and to come up with some viable solutions.

I finally succeed in confirming two major decisions. First, I will definitely dedicate the rest of my life to being a professional writer. I have always wanted to write on my own, and novels in particular, and now I will take the leap and *just do it*. I have written books of literary criticism and lots of ads and commercials, but this will be at a different level of creativity. This decision—which I have now confirmed definitively—originally dawned upon me a month or so earlier as a result of a stunning, life-changing epiphany, an incandescent confrontation with the Proverbial Light Bulb.

I am leaving the offices of the McCann Erickson ad agency in London after an interview. At that moment, I am pretty much tired of the whole advertising thing, it is freezing and pouring (*what, in London?*), and I am feeling afraid and shivering in my shoes and in no mood to whistle a happy tune. Standing outside the building just past the front entrance, I happen to look down at my feet, which are standing on the company's sacred motto inscribed in stone. I shuffle my feet back to be able to read the words, which say, TRUTH WELL TOLD. I chuckle to myself after reading this, because although the aphorism is pithy and clever, the "truth" is something that advertising often (to be kind) fudges. And I suddenly realize that I want to spend the rest of my life writing the truth, *my* truth. Yes, I will write stories and novels and essays that get to the essence of life and all its crucial issues, and I will tell them as well (and as enter-tainingly) as I possibly can. And it is at that point that I put this decision in motion, largely thanks to the 10,000-watt bulb switching on in my brain on that rainy day in London Town.

My second important decision is that I will move to a warm, sunny place, preferably near the ocean. The list of places I con-sider relocating to initially include my Top Ten of Rome, Ven-ice, Paris, Amsterdam, Stockholm, Boston, Philadelphia, San Francisco, San Diego, and Santa Barbara; the latter eventually wins out because of its beauty, climate, oceanic proximity, and tranquillity conducive to writing.

Well, one day toward the end of my stay, it is raining really hard (*what, in Florida?*) and I can't play tennis or golf, so on a whim, I decide to look up former major-league baseball player Frank Torre, who lives just a few doors down from my folks' house. My motivation, innocent and pure, is just to shmooz about baseball, a sport we both love dearly. (We were also both born in Brooklyn.) Frank is the older brother of Joe Torre, the former New York Yankees manager, and had a checkered career, highlighted by his two home runs in the 1957 World Series, in which his Milwaukee Braves defeated the Yankees.

So I ring him up.

"Hey, Frank, how ya doin'? Hope you don't mind my calling. My name is Bob Mitchell, and I'm only a few doors down visiting my folks and I love baseball and I've written and studied and thought about it a lot and I thought it'd be fun to sit and chat a while, seeing that it's raining."

Dead silence.

"Who's calling?"

"It's Bob Mitchell, and I'm only a few doors down—"

"Oh yeah, I got it. Sure, why not? Come on over. Say around two?"

"Two it is. See ya then."

Frank seems a bit withdrawn and perhaps suspicious (me calling him out of left field and all), but he is quite gracious, I am thinking, to accept my surprise self-invitation.

After I hang up, I suddenly realize that I have a fantastic, inspired, retroactively subliminal secondary motive for the visit: my dear friend Frank—another Frank!—Fleizach, whom I have known since our advertising days together in the 1980s, is, like me, an avid baseball fanatic and in fact the proud owner of an impressive collection of baseball memorabilia (magazines, yearbooks, paraphernalia, uniforms, baseballs, and the like). And so I decide to call him ASAP.

"Hey, asshole, whassup?"

We have employed this affectionate rectal reference with each other for decades as a badge of honor, a marker of both pride and humility. I even created an escutcheon for us that sports a pair of butt cheeks in the center, around which is inscribed ASS-HOLE SELECT SOCIETY (ASS) and under which is written NIHIL NISI LACUNA (Latin for "Nothing If Not a Cavity"), followed by LARCHMONT/SANTA BARBARA.

"*Asshole!*" Frank answers cheerily. "Great to hear from you. Nothing much. All good. Busy as usual. Whassup with you?"

"Listen, I need to ask you something. I seem to recall that you own a ball signed by Joe Torre, right?"

"Yep."

"Well, guess what. In about three hours, I'm going to be visiting his brother, Frank (great name, no?), and I thought you might like me to get him to sign a ball for your collection. You could put it in a plexiglass case right next to his brother's, and they could make a pretty classy pair of balls."

Frank guffaws, and I realize how that last sentence terminated.

"That would be *awesome* if you could pull it off!"

"I thought you might like the idea," I say. "Hopefully, I can get him to do it. Will keep you posted. Gotta run now to pick up a ball."

"Thanks, man, you're the best."

"Ditto."

So off I go to a local sporting goods store and pick up a cheapish Spalding hardball and bring it back home and put it in a shopping bag, along with a signed copy of my collection of sports stories, *How My Mother Accidentally Tossed Out My Entire*

Baseball-Card Collection, which I will sign and give to Frank as a token of my appreciation of his hospitality.

At the stroke of two, I am knocking at Frank Torre's door. He lets me in, offers me a coffee, and we begin to chat.

"First of all, Frank," I open, "many thanks for having me here. I love baseball, as I said, and I'm looking forward to our chat."

"No problem."

From the start, I become aware of two things: 1. Frank is a gracious and kindly man and 2. He also seems reserved and a bit uncomfortable. Could it possibly be because I foisted myself upon him unannounced? Or I am intruding on the privacy of a "public" person? Or he'd simply rather be alone?

Attempting to break the ice, I reach into my bag and pull out my signed book.

"Thought you might enjoy reading this. A little thing that was published a few years back—"

"Oh, thanks," Frank says pleasantly.

And then a dead silence.

I am feeling a bit uneasy with the (nonexistent) pace of the conversation, but I soldier on. We discuss baseball mostly, but also my heart bypass surgery in 1986 and his heart transplant in 1996 and then more baseball. It is slow going, and I'm having more than a little trouble drawing (and thawing) Frank out.

As luck would have it, I see in the distance, in the hallway, a series of maybe ten framed black-and-white photos of him and his various Braves teammates from the late fifties.

"Mind if I take a peek?" I ask, pointing to the pics.

"Sure, be my guest."

"But I am your guest *already*," I reply cleverly, hoping to evoke a smile.

Nothing.

We walk to the line of photos, and I recognize all of his fellow Braves.

"Hey, that's you with Billy Bruton . . . and Wes Covington . . . and Chuck Tanner . . . and Hammerin' Hank . . . and Del Crandall . . . and, wow, Eddie Mathews . . . and Johnny Logan . . . and Bob Buhl . . . and Lew Burdette . . . and ol' Spahnie . . ."

Talk about breaking the ice.

Presumably impressed by my knowledge of baseball back in the day, he loosens up a tad and puts on a semiforced smile as we reoccupy our living room seats, but the conversation is still a little stilted and halting. Something has to be done, and *now is the moment of truth*.

I reach into my bag and pull out the Spalding ball.

"Frank . . ."

I notice the glint of distress in his eyes, the moue about his lips, but I am way too resolute to be discouraged or to slow down now. I am on a Frigging Mission for the other Frank, and nothing is going to stop me.

"Listen," I continue, "I know you get this all the time, and I really wouldn't want to impose on you or to take advantage of my visit . . ."

Right.

". . . but . . ."

I compose my words punctiliously in my head.

". . . truth is, I have this friend. His name is Frank, too, and he would *so* love to have you sign this ball for him," I grovel obsequiously.

The deadest silence I've ever not heard. Frank has this glassy look, ostensibly immune to my plea.

I am officially becoming desperate, since I am on a Sacred Mission and have come this far, but my entreaty is apparently falling on deaf and oblivious ears.

I purse my lips, take a deep breath.

"And, you see, well, my friend Frank is ill . . ."

Nothing.

Frank Torre's face is blank and unmoved. I am now officially talking to a wall. I am beginning to panic. I hate lying with a passion, even a little white lie like this one, but I have no choice. *I must get this ball signed, or my goose is cooked.*

Beads of sweat are beginning to form on my forehead. I must do something stat, or else. And so, digging into my brain (or even lower) to pull out something even more impactful, I come up with a shameful embellishment of my last comment and blurt it hyperdramatically, as if the words were being artic-ulated by some method actor like Marlon Brando, John Garfield, or Rod Steiger:

". . . *very* ill . . ."

My devious intent, of course, is to throw out this line to suggest that my friend Frank (now the sick one!) is perhaps nearing the end, in the final stages of cancer or heart disease or some other nefarious assassin.

My embellishment must have somehow hit a nerve: Frank Torre abandons his comatose state, snaps to, snatches the base-ball out of my hands, pulls out a ballpoint from his pocket, and begins to inscribe the Spalding.

Oy.

I can see it coming, like a runaway freight train charging at me, gaining speed every second, and there is no way I can stop it. Before I can even make an attempt, it is all done, irrevocably, a fait accompli. The ball is signed, in ink no less, and there is not a blessed thing I can do about it. I know precisely what the ex-ballplayer has written on the ball, indelibly, and sure enough:

TO FRANK, GET WELL SOON! BEST, FRANK TORRE

To this very day, thanks to me and my idiotic (but well-meaning) gesture, my dear friend Frank Fleizach has this signed ball, prominently displayed in his memorabilia pantheon, to remind him forevermore of the dire, life-threatening illness he never had.

At the time, from desperation and loyalty, I had used a life-threatening illness as an excuse, a pretext, and, yes, a lie.

And now, ironically, it is I who am . . . *very* ill.

Back in the present, I am sitting at my desk and breathing a skosh more normally now, but I am still in serious doo-doo. My smile slowly evaporates from the fun of "The Torre Story," and my weary brain wanders, this time to a quote by the French philosopher Blaise Pascal: "The eternal silence of these infinite spaces terrifies me." *Why are we here on earth anyway, we infinitesimal specks of dust?* I am thinking. *Where do we fit in the Grand Scheme of things? Why does the universe get to live forever, and we mere mortals have to die, inevitably? Is the Unknown the source of all our fears?*

After my 25,693 days of existence here on Earth, is this the very moment my Life Membership Card is going to . . . *expire?*

3
Sleeping Policemen

In Jamaica, Belize, and Indonesia, speed bumps are wryly referred to as "sleeping policemen." Don't you *love* it?

We all encounter our fair share of these dormant cops during our lifetimes, but shortly after the stair-crawling episode, and still in April of 2015, I experience five real humdingers placed alarmingly and perilously close to one another.

I am in my writing study, Travis-picking on my Martin 000-28EC guitar, sipping a Balvenie fifteen-year-old single malt, surrounded by my books and framed artifacts, at utter peace with the universe.

Time to go pick up the mail. I descend the staircase, open the front door, and begin walking to the mailbox in (my daily) hopes that there is a royalty check and no bills today. I am halfway there, smack in the middle of the cul-de-sac and in full view of our neighbors. It is a typically gorgeous day, low seventies, no clouds, and I—

Bam!

Next thing I know, I am lying flat on my back, looking straight up at the sky, first in shock, then terror. *How the hell did*

I get here? Why am I lying on the ground, in the middle of the street? I must've passed out, because I have no memory of falling. Must've been a V-tach episode, I tell myself, *and my defibrillator must've shocked me to correct my arrhythmia. Yeah, that must be—*

Bam!

A second shock. This time, still lying on my back, I can feel it, like a large weight (oh, maybe 250 pounds?) has been dropped from the sky and onto my chest.

Moaning faintly, I attempt to pick myself up. No dice. Back on my back, I am now moaning deeply. Susan, ever vigilant, bolts out the front door, galloping to my rescue on her imaginary white stallion. She helps me up, and, draped on her strong shoulders, I limp to the curb. We rest there a few moments, I struggle to get back on my feet. A few minutes ago, I was down. But now, something's up.

Red flag time. We drive ASAP (Arrhythmia Suddenly A Problem) to the office of my cardiologist, who refers me to my electrophysiologist (defibrillator guy), who recommends a series of blood tests to evaluate the severity of the V-tach episode. He also recalibrates my defibrillator, hopefully to avoid further episodes.

The next week, I return to the crowded lab adjacent to nearby Scripps Memorial Hospital in Encinitas to have more blood drawn. Susan and I have been waiting in our chairs for, oh, maybe forty minutes. My name is finally called, and we approach the front desk area to—

Bam!

A third defibrillator attack. Like the first one, I am blasted into unconsciousness, transformed from vertical to horizontal, left by the electric current coursing through my body to lie on the floor, flat on my back, in the middle of the laboratory waiting room. If Susan hadn't been behind me to cushion my fall, I would almost certainly have cracked my skull open and expired on the spot.

Before I regain consciousness, the lab is cleared of patients, leaving only me, Susan, the techs, and the EMTs, who arrive to attend to me. All I remember of that mess is seeing Susan (the panic and love radiating simultaneously from her face), the EMTs loading me into an ambulance and carting me a few doors down to the hospital itself, a nurse connecting me to a bunch of IV drips, me throwing up all over myself and then falling into a deep sleep. I end up staying overnight at the hospital, after which I'm discharged to return home, a few red flags still flapping in the breeze but no white ones, which will never be waved by me or Susan.

The week after, I am in my writing study, as usual, beginning work on my fifth novel, which I decide will be all about—

Bam!

For the fourth time in three weeks, my defibrillator emits a shock, and I am propelled out of my chair and onto the floor.

As I am lying (and probably dying) there, I am flashing back to the time, about five years ago, when I almost drowned as a result of a similar defibrillator shock. Susan and I are visiting my older, daughter, Jenny, and her husband, Eric, at their lake house a few hours to the north of Atlanta. Hot day. Cold lake. *Bad combo.* Especially if you have a defibrillator inside your chest just begging to be shocked because of the thirty-five-degree temperature differential. Mea culpa: feeling frisky and desirous of escaping from the Georgian heat and humidity, I jump from the dock into the lake. The shock of it all is too much, and I begin to sink like a proverbial stone. As I continue to descend underwater, my fierce determination to live kicks in, and I somehow force myself to the surface, flapping my weakened arms like crazy, refusing to succumb to the attack. From the dock, Eric happens to see me floundering out of the corner of his eye, leaps into the water (he is much younger than I, immensely athletic and fit, and defibrillatorless), pulls my limp arms around his strong neck, and drags me to the ladder of the dock. After hyperventilating for a few minutes and clinging onto the ladder, I struggle up to the dock and lie there, gasping for air like a just-caught trout. From nowhere, a quote from legendary baseball executive Branch Rickey surfaces in my noggin:

> *Things worthwhile generally don't just happen . . . Good luck is what is left over after intelligence and effort have combined at their best . . . Luck is the residue of design.*

Am I a lucky bastard? No, attitude and desire and motivation (and Eric) are what saved me from drowning. I wanted to live, and I fought for it!

Funny, but the Latin words that are emblazoned on my high school insignia are Virtus Victrix Fortunae ("Character is the conqueror of chance"). I never thought about this too seriously back then, but now I am: be strong, be hopeful, be positive. And screw dumb luck!

Back in my Carlsbad study, I am lying on my back, still in a daze from the enormous electrical jolt that has just vaulted me here. Just a few seconds ago, I was writing notes furiously on my legal pad, happily inspired by the Muse, and now, here I am, inert and without—

Bam!

A fifth shock, and apparently this time I pass out for a scary while. When I come to, I look up and see Susan crouching over me, this relieved yet terrified look on her face. She relates to me how she found me here on the floor, not breathing and unconscious, and how she just performed emergency CPR on me as I lay unconscious, then called 911. And how at first I didn't respond to her efforts and she thought she had lost me forever, but eventually I began to breathe and to return to the land of the living. The EMT squad should be here any moment, she informs me with a quavering voice.

Two minutes later, the EMT people and the Carlsbad Fire Department paramedics arrive, bless their hearts. Eight men are surrounding me, two trying to prop me up in my chair. I am conscious once again and attempting to get my wits about me. I am half in denial and half barely aware of the goings-on, and my mind excuses itself from the room for a few brief seconds, time enough to mull over the rhythm of despair and joy in my life of seven decades.

My various achievements and joys flash through my mind: tennis rankings and tournament trophies; soccer scoring records; a year teaching in Angers, France, on a Fulbright Fellowship; teaching at Harvard, Purdue, and Ohio State; being an advertising creative director and winning creative awards; living and teaching commercial TV writing and production in Tel Aviv; living in France, Italy, the UK, Canada, and Sweden; writing ten published books, including three novels; giving the commencement address at Poly Prep, my high school alma mater; loving my great wife, Susan, and great kids and great friends and family and great life in California.

And yet, I am also thinking of my miserable failures and challenges: my mother "accidentally" tossing out my entire baseball-card collection just after I left home for college, having feelings of self-doubt and depression during my freshman year at college, enduring a difficult divorce, getting canned by an ad agency and being unemployed for a year, flailing around between careers deciding what to do next, all the heart crap I had to go through for the past thirty years.

A sarcastic (purported) quote by then-Ohio State assistant football coach Lou Holtz comes to mind: "The people of Columbus are great. They're behind you 100 percent, win or tie." And my fighting, competitive spirit kicks in. I'm gonna win this one! I've *gotta* win this one!

A ten-second memory now flashes through my mind, of a tennis match in the summer of 1960, the finals of the Camp Powhatan tournament, in Otisfield, ME. I am representing Camp Takajo (in Naples). It turns into a fiercely contested battle royal between the second seed (me) and the first seed (David Benjamin, who, later in life, ends up being the hugely successful and beloved tennis coach at Princeton). David is a wonderful player, and a really nice guy, too. He is the slight favorite, but, being an extremely competitive kid, I am going to will myself to upset him and battle to the finish and never give up and win if I have to kill myself to do it. Which I nearly do.

It is a steaming August day, maybe triple-figures steaming, and the match goes to a third set. In those days, there were no tie-breakers, and it seems that this final set will go on forever. At maybe 10-10, I am preparing to serve, and I feel that something is amiss. Terribly amiss. I look down at the handle of my Jack Kramer Autograph wooden racquet, and to my utter dismay, my right hand is stuck to the grip. Stuck, as in frozen solid due to dehydration. In digital agony, I walk to the bench at the side of the court and try to pry my fingers from the racquet, but to no avail. With the help of the Powhatan tennis and medical staffs, I am given a bottle of salt tablets, four of which I promptly gulp down.

Within minutes, I am back on the baseline serving, and I end up somehow fighting my way to an eked-out and satisfying victory.

With this winning thought buoying me in my ocean of fear, I am carted down the stairs by two EMT guys, my limp feet dragging behind me. I can't believe this is happening. Behind me, I hear the voice of Susan, who is praying for me to be okay and imploring me lovingly to hang in there. And then, inside my head, I hear the voice of Robert Frost reciting one of his clever couplets:

> *Forgive, O Lord, my little jokes on Thee*
> *And I'll forgive Thy great big one on me.*

Looking down at my temporarily crippled legs, I am thinking once again about Camp Takajo, where I spent seven glorious summers (from 1954 to 1960) between the ages of almost-ten and almost-sixteen. And, this time, about Freddie Eppsteiner.

This episode in my life embodies my first important encounter with illness and pain, albeit vicariously. Freddie was a cheery, likable kid who had one feature that distinguished him from us other 249 campers: he had contracted polio early in his life (presumably before Jonas Salk's vaccine had been developed) and wore cumbersome braces on his legs.

The first time I ever played in a baseball game with Freddie, I guess my reaction was the same as any other spoiled, unthinking, self-absorbed ten-year-old camper's: *How sad. What a shame. What a pity. Thank God it's not me!* As I watched Freddie clank his way down to first base, my own feelings of insulation and self-importance naturally surfaced. Feelings that were somewhat less than compassionate, even bordering on pity.

Freddie would rarely get on base. Once in a blue moon, he'd hit a slow roller to the left side that the third sacker would throw wildly, way over the first baseman's head and deep into the woods and behind some blackberry bush. By the time it was retrieved and finally chucked back to the bag, he'd barely beat it out by a whisker, causing the guilt-ridden infielder who made the error to hang his head in ignominious shame.

And shame is what I, ten-year-old idiot that I was, must have felt until I realized the amazing heroism of this kid. Just imagine: he was thrust into a situation where he was surrounded by a group of basically decent athletes, some even extremely gifted. And all "normal." But what was so incredible was his good cheer. Well aware of the "unlevel playing field" caused by his handicap, he would limp his way to first base time after time, hunching up his shoulders to give himself some inertia (and perhaps to absorb Lord knows what pain), braces clanging, head jerking back, arms flailing. *And a frigging smile on his face!*

Truth is, even though I never told him (I wish I had) and even though he'd never known it (I wish he had), I came to admire and respect Freddie in a special way I never felt with any other athlete before or since. And what I most respected, in those innocent days under the sweet-smelling Maine pines, was his desire. More than anyone else, Freddie seemed just to want to be playing the game. Not to be victorious, as we others did, pushed by some Western, goal-oriented "achievement" ethic. Not to please someone else (parents? counselors? older sibling?). But simply to play, to participate, *to be there.*

Freddie's desire was never more evident (I find it somewhat frightening that I still remember the incident so vividly to this day) than in the 1956 version of the Annual Camp Takajo Soda Pop Baseball Game, or ACTSPBG.

In those days of nonpermissiveness, discipline, and privation, the summer camp environment was in fact closer to that of a boot camp. There were strict rules of conduct, one of which was that under no circumstances was any candy or ice cream or soda pop permitted on the premises (except when snuck in by liberal and iconoclastic counselors). With the exception of the weekly "candy sale," at which time you were allowed to purchase one single solitary candy bar. (The most popular candy in those days were Charleston Chews, Bonomo's Turkish Taffy, 3 Musketeers, Clark Bars, and—a distant fifth—Zagnut. For the record, my personal fave was Power House.) Even during Visiting Day, parents were told in no uncertain terms that candy, ice cream, and soda were strictly forbidden as "bunk gifts." Of course, in their nurturing zeal, they rarely listened, and the clandestine transgression of this particular draconian law was rampant.

Oh, yeah. The ACTSPBG . . .

Anyway, because of the strict "no-sugar" laws, it was a game to which every camper looked forward eagerly. Here's how it went down: when it was your turn, you marched up to the plate and faced a "good-control" pitcher (obviously, a counselor), so walks and boredom weren't factors, and took your cuts. In the first- and third-base coaching boxes were positioned twenty-something waiters from the mess hall, in whose strong arms were nestled serving trays filled with Daisy paper cups and a number of bottles of assorted sparkling, sugary beverages (diet soda did not become available for at least another few years): Coca-Cola, Nedick's orange soda, Hires Root Beer. Why the game was so popular and anticipated every summer had everything to do with the system of reward in this environment of privation: if you got a single, the waiters served you a cup of soda; a double, you got two cups; a triple, three; and a homer would allow you to gulp down an entire bottle, to the envy and dismay of your teammates and opponents alike. If you didn't reach base, you were rewarded with absolutely zippo. Talk about motivation!

My memory of these games that is most vivid is the time when Freddie comes up to the plate and, to the surprise of virtually everyone on the field (and off: word travels fast in camp), gets hold of a fat one and just *creams* it. I mean, he gets every inch of it, the way I'd never seen him get hold of one before. And, a smile on his face as always, he hobbles off to first and, realizing the ball is still traveling down the rocky road beyond left field and past two bunks (Illinois and Iroquois), stops briefly in shock before making his way to second. *Second!* Freddie's even contemplating reaching second base is like America's contemplating sending a man to the moon in the mid-'50s. But reach it he does, in plenty of time to beat the throw, which at long last makes its way, via two or three relay men, to second base. I recall that for a split second, Freddie actually considers trying for third but, appreciating the already-prodigious feat of doubling and not wanting to tarnish its memory, must have thought better of it and remains frozen to the bag. At this point, it transpires as in a movie: as if in slow motion, campers begin, one by one, to applaud, until everyone is paying tribute to Freddie's feat (and feet). As the applause reaches a crescendo, the waiter (it was Arnie Abrams, if memory serves) trots out to give him his just desserts, the two cups of pop. And a huge ear-to-ear smile fills up Freddie's face. He has accomplished the impossible, and in the ACTSPBG, no less!

Ever since, I have especially appreciated several aspects of athletic competition (and life) more than I ever would have had I not seen Freddie Eppsteiner perform on a baseball diamond. Never give up. Keep on trying, no matter what the odds and how great the challenge. Be true to your inner voice through all the ups and downs that might befall you. Pressure? *What pressure?* And, finally, as you run down that first-base line of life, keep smiling. Oh, above all, keep smiling.

I have never forgotten that image of Freddie, and the memory of his disability and his tenacity is adding not only much-needed perspective to what I am experiencing now as I am ushered out the front door, feet dragging on the ground, and placed in the ambulance, but, nearly as important, a faint smile to my face.

As I settle down in the ambulance, my fuzzy brain summons up a few mushy quotes from Romantic poets (Keats, Lamartine) about the heart. I love poetry, but now, as I recite the verses in my head, the words seem particularly hollow. Yeah, fine for those guys to warble about the wondrous beating of a heart in love, in ecstasy, feeling joy. To sing about this organ as if it were an abstraction, a reservoir of spirituality and soulfulness. But now is not the time, and I am chiding myself for all the mushiness I have just summoned: *Get real, man! All the heart does is beat and circulate blood to the rest of the body. That's all it is, a pump!*

And right now, mine—pistons, valves, gaskets, O-rings, cylinder housings, intake manifolds, shaft bearings, and all—is in dire need of a freaking Master Plumber.

4
Those Two Impostors

Of all the scariest thoughts a person can have, the idea of being put on life support is, in my opinion, right up there.

I am admitted (again) to Scripps Memorial Hospital in Encinitas, CA, and immediately hooked up to a series of life-support IV drips: principally milrinone and dobutamine to improve heart function, plus bumex and lasix, nitroglycerine, insulin, heparin, delaudid, vancomycin, and other assorted pharmaceutical goodies. I am informed that my defibrillator has shocked me twelve times in all and that, because of the serious arrhythmias, my heart is unable to function on its own without these medications.

I am poked and prodded and undergo a ferocious barrage of tests to determine whassup: ultrasounds, x-rays, biopsies, CT and PET scans, angiograms, blood work, you name it.

I feel like crap.

After two weeks, I am moved to two other hospitals, first Scripps Green and then Scripps La Jolla. More IVs, more x-rays, more biopsies, more scans, more blood work, more everything. Then more of the same.

As the witch's brew of pain, boredom, anxiety, ignorance, and panic continues to bubble up within me, accompanied by plenty of toil and trouble, Dr. Ajay Srivastava, my new cardiologist and heart failure specialist, strides confidently into my room one day. He is smart, congenial, and direct and looks at me with a warm twinkle in his eye. He explains to me in detail my condition, and what the options might be, with just the right combination of diplomacy, optimism, and caution. They need to do more tests to determine the next steps and the best treatment with the best chances of positive results.

And then, to my delight, we engage in a stimulating conversation about a topic dear to my now-troubled heart.

"So, Mr. Mitchell—"

"Actually, Ajay, this has always bothered me. I never really liked the idea of people addressing me as 'Mr.'"

"So why is that?"

"Well, it's sort of a long story. My dad was an MD, a pathologist, so people always called him 'Dr.' As a kid, I respected that title. Then, when I went to college, I was kind of nudged by Dad to be premed, you know, in those days there was that generational baton-passing thing, but it didn't work out because my left brain doesn't function all that well and I didn't 'get' organic chemistry and the first day of freshman chem, I pulled out my lab drawer too hard and nearly everything in it crashed to the floor—Erlenmeyer flasks, pipettes, test tubes—to the tune of about two hundred bucks worth of paraphernalia."

Ajay smiles and emits a polite chuckle.

"Then I earned a PhD in French literature and the title of 'Dr.' But I was a little schizophrenic about it. I liked having a title that reflected how hard I had worked to earn it, but on the other hand, I didn't like the aspect of being separated, segregated from all the 'Mr.'s out there. So I shied away from using it most of the time, except when I had little kids of my own, and when I went to the movies, for instance, I instructed the babysitter to call the theater if there was an emergency, but to be sure to page 'Dr. Mitchell,' which would add urgency and gravitas to her request."

"I get it," Ajay says after I am finished with my diatribe. "And now, do you go by 'Dr.'?"

"Actually, in the end, I'm not really fond of titles at all. I much prefer to avoid 'Dr.' and 'Mr.' and 'Ms.' and 'Mrs.' So I call everyone by their first names, which is way more personal and cuts through all the bullshit of titles and stature."

"I don't disagree with you . . . Bob." Obviously, this smart doc gets it.

"That's cool . . . Ajay. Oh, and as far as 'real' doctors go, I feel comfortable calling them by their first names and like them to do the same to me. The one place I have had trouble with this, though, is at their offices."

"Meaning?"

"Meaning I'll be in a doctor's office, and I'll say to the receptionist or nurse, 'Excuse me, is John running late today?' And she'll say to me, 'Yes, Dr. Smith is running a bit late.' And I'll say, 'Well, I understand, John is a busy guy.' And she'll say, 'Yes, Dr. Smith has a lot of patients.' Well, you get my drift."

"You know, I don't disagree with you," Ajay points out. "It's a tough one. In the end, we live in a meritocracy, so it's okay to be proud of what you have accomplished and the degrees you've earned."

"Totally," I agree. "And the other side of the coin is hubris, because lots of doctors—academics and physicians alike—feel a certain haughtiness about the whole thing and like to feel that they are in a way superior to people who don't have advanced degrees, and that, I think, places them on a pedestal, especially in the eyes of the people working for them, and it creates an unfortunate distance, even a chasm, between doctors and nondoctors!"

Dr. Srivastava, I mean Ajay, is a *mentsh* of the first order and a pleasure to chat with, and I am feeling not quite so wretched after our lively little exchange.

When he leaves, though, my mood is less ebullient, and I am thinking about the years of hard work I spent earning my doctorate all those decades ago, but so what? Here I am on life support, my future existence up in the ozone, so what the hell good has it done me? Is the concept of "success" an illusion? Is "failure" in life inevitable?

I am seeing in my mind's eye a couplet from Rudyard Kipling's poem "If." I am envisioning it because I have read the poem many times and seen it inscribed on the wall above the players' entrance to Centre Court at Wimbledon, and because it fits the occasion perfectly:

> *If you can meet with Triumph and Disaster*
> *And treat those two impostors just the same . . .*

Kipling sure got *that* one right. Are winning and losing impostors perhaps because each pretends to be an end in itself? Is the truth not closer to the fact that the two complement each other, functioning in relation to each other's necessity? To use a sports metaphor, a bad bounce, a line call, an inch one way or the other can technically separate a winner from a loser. But perseverance and total effort and passion are the great barometers of character, and no bounce or call or near-miss can define who you are inside—win *or* lose—if you keep on trying.

I am thinking about how we Americans tend to be obsessed with winning, success, and achievement. This drive is everywhere apparent, from success in business to victory in Iraq to triumphing in sports. I could write a book about it. (In fact, I have.)

I am recalling with a chuckle George Brett's quip, "If tying is like kissing your sister, losing is like kissing your grandmother with her teeth out."

Sure, a healthy desire to excel and to achieve is admirable, even crucial. But the longer I live, the more I learn that failure and losing are not really negatives, but integral parts of life and, strangely enough, necessary ones that give winning and success a context and a deeper, fuller meaning. And more than winning, losing forces us to learn important life lessons, to improve ourselves, to be prepared for the next time. I cannot possibly believe any more in this concept than I already do.

In fact, lying alone in my hospital bed and attached to all my IV drips, I am actually recollecting an incident that happened twenty years before on the tennis court, when *losing actually saved my life*. Literally. Me, the toughest *hombre* in these here parts!

It is 1995, and, newly moved to Berkeley from the East and recently divorced and having just turned fifty and starting my life anew, I am at the Chabot Canyon Racquet Club in

Oakland, CA, playing in my very first senior tennis tournament ever. The week before, I had played a really close match there against former baseball superstar second baseman Joe Morgan, and I am in tip-top shape. Joe has a high ranking in the Western Seniors, as I recall, so I figure I have a decent chance to go deep in the tourney.

In the opening round, during a match that I am dominating against a crafty and unpredictable lefty baseliner, I run furiously to retrieve a drop shot, and suddenly something doesn't feel quite right. I am feeling weak and a little more out of breath than I should be, but I shrug it off and barely make it through the next point. I am up two breaks of serve in the opening set, 5-2, and there's no way I can lose this match and no way I will let my little physical sleeping policeman stop me from doing so.

On the changeover, I am catching my breath and gulping down some Gatorade and feeling discomfort in my jaw and even a little nauseated, then pain in my chest and also down my left arm. Classic symptoms of a myocardial infarction. Been there, done that. At first, I am in denial. I have been symptomless ever since my emergency quadruple-bypass surgery nine years before, at Montefiore Medical Center in the Bronx. I mutter to myself, *Nothing's wrong. Let's take care of business and wrap up this match. Keep on fighting through this, no matter what.* At which point an imaginary crimson-colored, hornèd Devil with a tail appears on my left shoulder and an imaginary dressed-in-white, wingèd Angel with a halo appears on my right one, each apparition giving me counsel via the closest available ear.

D: "Don't you even *think* of stopping now. What are you, a coward? A quitter? A wuss? You wait fifty years to enter your first senior tournament, and then you just give up? What, you get a little itty-bitty pain in your chest, and you wave the freaking white flag?"

A: "Dear soul, I know how hard it is for you to stop playing and default, but for the love of God you must, because something dire is about to befall you."

D: "You gonna listen to that goody-goody with the sissy halo? Listen, nothin's wrong with you, and you know it. You got this guy by the short and curlies, so why don't you just be a man and grow a pair and squash him like the bug that he is?"

A: "I beg you to stop now and take care of yourself. You are a worthy, loving, caring, and creative being, and we need you here on Earth."

D: "How sappy can you get? I mean, man, gimme a break. Speaking of which, you have *two* breaks, and it won't take much more to polish this total loser off."

A: "I will pray for you and hope that you will love yourself enough to leave the court now and get some help. God bless."

Too proud to quit, I decide to bite the bullet, take my medicine, and grit it out. But the pain in my chest is hindering my play, and how. I am not the same player I was in the opening seven games, not even close to being the same person. My body is a stranger, and I am running on fumes and pure heart (which is now racing). But I decide to soldier on, of course. Because I believe in never giving up. Because I am a proud and fierce competitor. Because I am a *total and complete moron.*

And the harder I fight, the more I hurt, and the more I lose: 5-2 quickly becomes 5-5, then 5-6. At the changeover, I am seriously considering listening to my inner angel and defaulting.

But it is a struggle: my heart, which wants to fight on, vs. my head, which wants no part of that and thinks it would be stupid. I feel deep down that I should listen to my head, but my heart and my instincts are acting like out-of-control jerks. My thinking is that I should really default now, because even if, by miracle, I should make it to the tie-breaker and win it, reason dictates that there's no way on Earth I can win another set, much less another game. It is hopeless, pointless. But despite this rational argument, for now, my heart wins out.

Somehow, I win the twelfth game, and we go into a tie-breaker. But I had put so much energy into winning that last game that I have little left and drop the breaker, 7-2.

Slumping on the bench before the start of the second set, I am feeling a little dizzy and am debating with myself, but the debate is short-lived. Despite my competitive drive, I know the jig is up, and I finally come to my senses and realize the seriousness of my condition. I simply can't continue, because if I do, something bad will certainly happen. And so, uncharacteristically (I've never defaulted a match before or after or ever), I do the unthinkable: before it is too late, I walk over to my opponent, shake his hand, and say, begrudgingly, "Can't go on. Sorry. Nice match." Just in the nick of time, as the doc in a nearby hospital—who informs me I had suffered a mild heart attack—tells me not long after. Had I not come to my senses after losing the first set and continued playing, it would probably have been game, set, match against my survival.

Competition, in its own way, was teaching me lessons that I knew all too well but, in the heat of the moment, was slow to acknowledge. Know your limits. Give it everything you've got, but when you have nothing left to give, don't be a shmuck, give it up. Or maybe, the hard way, it was asking me to respect that double dose of reality, those twin pearls of classical wisdom that the Delphic oracle had dispensed over two millennia ago and that are still exquisitely true: "*Meden agan, gnothi seauton*," "Nothing in excess, know thyself."

Returning to my hospital room reality, I am thinking about how much losing can help us learn. My eyes are focusing on all my IV drips, the monitor, the tubes, the needles stuck into my right arm. And then, suddenly, like a pot of water that has just reached the boiling point, my fierce competitive nature bubbles up, and I am determined to survive my current challenge, to *win* this one, goddammit. Screw Kipling. After all, this is the seventh game of the World Series, and there's no tomorrow. Except, that is, if I beat the odds.

So here's the deal. Tomorrow, after all these tests and all this time, I am scheduled to have an LVAD (a left ventricular assist device, a heart pump with very heavy and unwieldy external batteries) inserted inside my chest. It is not something I want to do. Not at all. It will be horribly inconvenient, for me and for Susan. The tube coming out of my body and the equipment to which it is attached will have to be cleaned often, the batteries in the power pack recharged often, the twenty pounds of batteries will have to be lugged around with me in two pouches wherever I go (and, as an added bonus, I will only be able to wear loose-fitting shirts). Susan and I have taken preliminary maintenance lessons in my room from the lovely and knowledgeable clinical coordinator, Lauren Wolman, about how to clean it and turn it on and off and have absorbed a great number of rules, regulations, and caveats. The worst thing about the LVAD is that it is meant to be a temporary bridge to a transplant; but if they implant it now, I'll probably have to have it in my chest until the end of my life, since it will be at least a year before they can do another invasive chest surgery (my body will have to recover during that time from this one), and by that time, I'll be past the accepted maximum age eligibility for a transplant. So I guess you could say (if you dare) that I'm between a rock and a heart place.

At the last minute, the executive committee miraculously comes to the rescue, having the foresight and wisdom to decide that, as risky as it would be, a transplant would in fact be a far better option for me at my "advanced age" and with my heart in such wretched condition. Thank you, Ajay and colleagues! *How many bullets can I dodge?* I ask myself. (Little do I know the imminence and quantity of projectiles about to be aimed at my heart.)

After I receive the cheery transplant news from the committee, I am sitting alone in my bed (Susan has, sadly, left for home) and contemplating the concept of "Plan B" (the strategy, not the morning-after pill). And thinking about planning ahead and being flexible and having an alternative and handy backup strategy. About focusing on a single path, but also anticipating something going wrong or changing that necessitates a shift in direction.

Which has been known to happen in life.

I am musing on the game of chess, and particularly on the incomparable Bobby Fischer (the nonpareil chess champion, not the execrable human being). About how he not only had a

Plan B for every move, but a Plan C, a Plan D, a Plan X. How great chess players have the ability and the vision to see far ahead, anticipating their opponents' possible options.

It is now 1989 in my mind. I am harking back to a creative presentation I am making to one of my advertising clients, Tumi, now a world-renowned top-quality bags and luggage company. (I always loved that their name referred to a Peruvian ceremonial knife.)

The assigned black-and-white print ad is for one of their products, the Stowaway Tote, which is to be offered free of charge with the purchase of one of Tumi's other fine products. A sort of "Buy One, Get a Different One Free" ad.

It was always my habit, when I presented ads to the company's advertising and marketing department, to have a "Plan B." They were a tough bunch of guys, very literal, extremely sensitive to any "negative" reference even if it was obviously meant to elevate their product, not very sensitive to my wry and tongue-in-cheek brand of humor, not too receptive to the entertainment value of an ad (which always makes the "sell" more palatable and powerful). In other words, pretty typical clients. And so I always brought two ads to the meetings, one I loved and one I sorta liked but that was definitely my second choice. My typical M. O. was to enter the room, place my first choice (Plan A) on the conference table, and furtively slip my second choice (Plan B) on the floor and under my chair, just in case. And every time with this client—without exception—my preferred ad was rejected, and my Plan B was then scooped off the floor, presented, and, of course, approved with wild enthusiasm.

But this time is different. I have decided before the meeting to hoodwink and bamboozle my clients by perpetrating the ol' switcheroo and presenting the ad I sorta liked first, with my Plan A ad, waiting hungrily to be presented and bought, on the floor. I am pretty excited about my Plan A on this day and can't wait to race through the lukewarm Plan B ad first, which of course will be rejected summarily, and get to my preferred one.

My (preferred) Plan A ad features two images, one on top of the other. The one on top is a map of the USSR (this was at the time of *glasnost*—Gorbachev's policy of "openness"—and a few years before the Soviet Union was dissolved), and the one on the bottom is the handsome Tumi Stowaway Tote. The headline below reads, ONE OF THESE IS NOW FREE. The final line of body copy is "Offer not valid in Leningrad or Omsk."

Needless to say, Plan B is unanimously approved immediately, amid deafening cheers and applause. The clients love it so much, in fact, that they refuse to entertain any other alternative offerings—such is their unwavering satisfaction with the Plan B ad—while my beloved Plan A ad sits lonely and neglected and unopened beneath my chair. (The happy ending: Plan B doesn't enjoy too much success, and Plan A is eventually bought, runs in the papers, and increases sales.)

I am told that tomorrow, I will be transferred to Cedars-Sinai Hospital in LA and hopefully, after I am thoroughly checked out, put on the waiting list to get a brand-new heart.

Which is making me think of LA and all the time I have spent in that crazy, lunatic, ultrafunky city. Homeless people peeing in the streets. People of all ages shooting up smack on the curbs. The abominable traffic jams. The slummy sections and the fancy-shmancy ones. The great concerts in the Hollywood Bowl. The superb restaurant scene. Shooting TV commercials there for more than a decade, and luxuriating (free of charge) at the Mondrian and the Four Seasons. Buying antique earrings to bring home to my daughters, Jenny and Sarah, at Retail Slut (so LA!) on Melrose when they were kids.

And Cedars-Sinai and its unparalleled reputation. And already having been there for various surgeries and checkups for my defibrillator, performed by the talented (and charming) electrophysiologist, Dr. Michael Shehata. And recovering from defibrillator surgery in March of 2011, the same day that Elizabeth Taylor died there of congestive heart failure. (By the way, her death was announced in all the papers around the world the next day; incxplicably, my surgery wasn't.)

I am filled with the contradictory feelings of first anxiety and then hope in anticipation of my transplant. First, *Think about it: having someone else's heart beating inside your chest!* And then, *Think about it: having someone else's heart beating inside your chest!*

As far as the anxiety is concerned, well, who could blame me? My first reaction to the news is emotional. My old heart, close to death, will be tossed in the garbage and left to rot there. This heart that has been with me, dutifully pumping my blood for over seventy years, will be with me no more.

I had heard about a book written a while ago by the dancer Claire Sylvia in which she claims that she took on the characteristics of her heart donor. I am, however, skeptical about that (although I am a romantic at heart and have been known to cry during sappy movies), because, again, the heart—as we all know—is just a pump! The first image that comes to mind

in the midst of my transplant anxiety is that of Marty Feldman playing Igor in Mel Brooks's movie *Young Frankenstein*. Of
course, the idea of a brain transplant is clearly a fantasy, since
it will probably never be attempted (but . . . what do I know?).
I am imagining, instead, Marty sneaking into the lab in Tran-
sylvania and grabbing the jar with my new *heart* in it and dropping it and it crashes to the floor and then he takes another
jar, this time one containing an abnormal heart—a twisted, evil
heart!—and it is shipped to Cedars-Sinai and then it is inserted
into my chest and then . . .

And then, the hope. Ah, the wonders of technology and
of science! Just imagine: in a nutshell, they take a heart from
someone who is clinically still alive but brain-dead, pack it in
ice, fly it to the hospital, then they take my sick old heart out of
my body, put the new one in, and sew it to my various veins and
arteries. And then, all of a sudden—*Abracadabra!* and *Shazam!*—
I am alive again and breathing normally and full of energy and
appetites and stamina. And hope.

I've often thought to myself that everyone on Earth should
be deeply grateful that the technological progress of civilization
never depended on me. Otherwise, we would almost certainly
be living back in the prewheel days.

5

Last Leaf

What could Cole Porter have been thinking when he was writing his classic song "You're the Top"? Sure, he compared the object of his affection to all manner of superlatives: the Coliseum, the Louvre museum, a symphony by Strauss, a Bendel bonnet, a Shakespeare sonnet, Mickey Mouse, the Nile, the Tower of Pisa, the smile on the Mona Lisa, Mahatma Gandhi, Napoleon brandy, a summer night in Spain, the National Gallery, Garbo's salary, cellophane, turkey dinner, the Derby winner, an Arrow collar, a Coolidge dollar, Fred Astaire's feet, an O'Neill drama, Whistler's mama, camembert, a rose, Dante's Inferno, Durante's nose, a dance in Bali, a hot tamale, an angel, a Botticelli, Keats, Shelley, Ovaltine, a boom, the dam at Boulder, the moon over Mae West's shoulder, a Waldorf salad, a Berlin ballad, the boats on the Zuider Zee, an old Dutch master, Lady Astor, broccoli, romance, the steppes of Russia, and the pants on a Roxy usher. But how could he have omitted Cedars-Sinai Medical Center's Advanced Heart

Disease Center from his laundry list of laudatory lyrics? Maybe it had too many syllables.

Cedars-Sinai is in fact the Mecca of heart transplant hospitals. It is the trailblazer for the procedure worldwide, performs annually more heart transplants than any other hospital, and has a 91 percent rate of success for patients living more than a year after transplant. In short, it is *the* place to be if you need a new ticker. Especially if you are over seventy: this hospital is known to accept people of this age, while most other hospitals will not. Yet despite all this, the challenges about to confront me will be immense (duh-uh).

I am still on life support (the same IV drips as at Scripps). Endless biopsies, x-rays, ultrasounds, blood work, angiograms, EKGs, scans. Ad infinitum, it appears.

As phenomenal as this hospital is, as talented and caring as the staff and team of cardiologists and surgeons are, and as fortunate as I am to be here, at this time in my life and as my heart continues to hang on for dear life, well, to be frank, paradise it ain't.

In fact, weeks crawl by filled with pain, boredom, mental angst, and unthinkably bad food, and I spend many hundreds of hours staring out my window and meditating. Everything is happening in slow motion, as if it were shot overcranked at 120 frames per second. The uncertainty about whether I will be eligible for a new heart seems certain, and the wait to determine whether I will end up with one seems endless.

Not to complain (don't you love that ludicrous rhetorical lie?), but to add to my anguish, my room is depressing (small, dark, plus fluorescent lighting), and my average day is filled with lovely distractions: peeing every hour on the dot into a plastic urinal to be measured for volume, rolling my unwieldy monitor into the bathroom with the help of a nurse while wires twist uncooperatively around my bed, taking short walks in the hallways barely able to hold myself up and out of breath and being forced to return to my room after three minutes tops, being awakened from a rare nap by the not-so-faint moans of pain from all the adjoining rooms . . .

I receive regular visits from a barrage of cardiologists, fellows, residents, social workers, physical therapists, psychiatrists, endocrinologists, nephrologists, pulmonologists, and infectious disease docs, plus a new RN every twelve hours. Every single hour, I am poked, prodded, interviewed, interrogated, pushed, pulled, stretched, examined, tested, and injected. Each member of the cardiology team explains to me, often and in no uncertain terms, that these tests and exams and interviews, this thoroughness to the nth degree, are absolutely necessary, all having the common and collective goal of demonstrating beyond a shadow of a shadow of a shadow of a doubt that I am an irrefutably deserving physical and mental recipient, a perfect candidate to be placed on the 1A (preferred) waiting list for a new heart, all vital and crucial and sine qua nons because of my age and because there are way more transplant candidates out there (and in here) than there are available hearts to divvy up amongst us.

Despite (and because of) all this, I am hanging in there, still immensely hopeful, still trying to focus on the positive. Yet— paradoxically—I am exhausted, in ineffable pain, running out of patience, bored out of my cranium, and anxious about the future. It ain't easy, but then again, nothing is ever easy in life.

And then, there is the straw-that-bent-but-didn't-quite-break the patient's back (and front): the total lack of privacy and of personal dignity. That's just the way it is waiting for a heart during a long hospital stay. People watching over you, intruding on you (all for your own good, mind you), interrupting, prying, just doing their jobs. Your private parts, for starters, are no longer private. Now they are your *public* parts. (This reminds me, as I write, of the very first scholarly article I ever proofread as managing editor of a large academic publication, the *French Review*. The original, misprinted title of this article about the great French poet Rimbaud—which, of course, I promptly corrected—read, "Arthur Rimbaud's Private and Pubic Image.") Catheters are inserted and removed, exams are performed, gowns are removed and replaced, sponge (actually towel) baths are given. What's more, your bodily functions are no longer private functions (private seatings, you might say) to which only you are invited. Now, they are basically ONP: Open to the Nursing Public.

One day, in the midst of my misery, a young (thirtysomething) man in blue scrubs enters my room. Forget about Raymond: *Everybody Loves Dael.*

With his boyish smile, mischievous look, rogue wisp of hair across his forehead, and professional caring and self-assuredness, Dr. Dael Geft is a cross between Huck Finn and Martin Arrowsmith. He is a true *mentsh*, a regular guy but so much more (this is the proper spelling and translation, according to Leo Rosten, preeminent Yiddish guru), and one of the cardiologists who, no matter who you speak to in the hospital, is universally admired and loved.

We spend twenty minutes or so chatting, which to me is amazing in light of his busy schedule of rounds, surgical procedures, and consults. What is so important to me is not only his caring, but also the fact that I have someone whom I like and can relate to during this challenging time in my life. Dael is patient, answers all my (many) questions, is really smart (like all the docs at Cedars-Sinai), and has a keen sense of humor. He is also quite skilled at instilling confidence in me, but at the same time at being a realist. After going through my numbers and test results, he tells me, to my delight and relief, "You're going to be okay, Bob. I am certain that ultimately we'll get a new heart for you. You're strong mentally. You have a great attitude, and you deserve it. But be patient, because we have to check you out thoroughly for everything. Lots of ups and downs. And that'll take a little time."

I also think that our both being Jewish and the fact that he is a Sabra (a native Israeli) and I spent a year in Tel Aviv in 1994 in some way helped bond us with this special connection.

Toward the end of our chat, I feel comfortable enough with him to recount a story of me and the Hebrew language, out of which I think he'll get a kick.

As the story goes, I spend almost all of 1994 in Israel teaching and lecturing on advertising creativity, conceptual writing, and commercial TV film writing and production at three ad agencies in Tel Aviv, as well as lecturing on art direction, design, and creative commercial writing at the Bezalel Academy of Arts and Design in Jerusalem.

By the end of my first few weeks in Tel Aviv, I have settled into my little flat on the Rehov Pinsker (thanks to the generosity of the Gitam ad agency), just a few blocks from the popular Dizengoff Circle, where a few days after I leave Israel for good in mid-October, a Hamas bomb set off in a bus kills twenty-two civilians and wounds fifty.

It has become my habit, on the way home after a day's work at Gitam, to stop at a stand right next to my flat and purchase a bag of *botnim* (peanuts) and a bottle of single-malt Scotch. Back in my flat, I would sit on the balcony, nursing my Scotch and munching my peanuts, and look across the street and watch Israelis walking and talking, civilians and soldiers alike. Directly across from me is a little store above which hangs a green awning with four letters printed on it:

$$ |6| \delta $$

As I continue to look at the awning and take another sip of my amber ambrosia, I become curious as to why this particular store is named "Ibid." After a few minutes of pondering, I conclude that these Israelis must be terribly well-educated people (which I already know), because they know their Latin well: they named this store "Ibid" because in Latin, *ibidem* means "in the same place" (Ibid. is used in endnotes of academic papers to mean "ditto," or the same source as in the previous note). And since I had seen other green awnings in town with the same word written on them, I reason that this is a chain of stores that sell the same product(s).

A week later, I am sipping my Scotch and eating my peanuts on my balcony and looking at the same green awning, and it suddenly occurs to me that, no, I was mistaken and perhaps these Israelis aren't so classically educated and the name of the store is in fact "Ibis," which, maybe, just maybe, is the national bird of Israel:

וֹוֹ6

A few days later, I am sipping my tawny nectar and eating my salty legumes on my balcony and looking at the same green awning, and I finally realize—duh-uh—that I have been a nincompoop all this time. When I first arrived in Israel, and maybe it was due to jet lag or disorientation, I was not really thinking in Hebrew when I saw the written language—which, from time to time, resembles certain English letters. So what I saw as "Ibid" and "Ibis" was the result of my reading left to right, whereas Hebrew is, of course, to be read right to left. And so, at long last coming to my senses and with my vestigial knowledge of the Hebrew alphabet (it was not since my bar mitzvah thirty-seven years before that I had been immersed in the written language), I finally read the sign correctly, right to left:

וֹ6וֹוֹ

And I realize that the letters are actually spelling out the word L-O-T-O. The awnings explain that in all these identical stores in town, *people can buy Lotto tickets!*

I show Dael the Hebrew letters, which I had scribbled on an index card, and he laughs his charming laugh, and the Jewish doctor-Jewish patient bond affixes itself to us. His smile, unlike that of most of my dad's medical colleagues I grew up knowing through his practice (and, sadly, a number of physicians practicing today), reveals—lo and behold—*a bedside manner!*

Dael is one of a team of amazing cardiologists at the Cedars-Sinai Advanced Heart Disease Center whom I will get to know in time (the others: Jon Kobashigawa, Jignesh Patel, Michele Hamilton, Michelle Kittleson, David Chang, Jaime Moriguchi, Mamoo Nakamura, Larry Czer, Babak Azarbal, and Antoine Hage), which was a great comfort to me as the days dragged on and I met one daunting challenge after another. I was constantly appreciative of their solicitousness, their caring, and their ability to keep my spirits up with a smile or a gesture or an encouraging word. In their largely left-brained universe crowded with trilettered and technical acronyms like RNA, PAP, MCI, ICM, MRI, CBC, CHF, CAD, RCC, EKG, RCA, and LAD, there was, somehow, always time for a little TLC and LOL.

In fact, the power of positive thinking is one of the most potent, unprescribed, over-the-counter, free-of-charge medicines available! In my situation, added to my congenital positivity and optimism, it quite possibly meant the difference between life and death. Of course, the cardiologist's primary job is to diagnose, to examine, to quantify, to explicate, and, in its purest state, to be alchemists, turning the lead (or worse!) of pathology into the gold of good health. But, especially from my patient's point of view, an equally essential part of their job description should be as transporters and disseminators of hope, empathy, compassion, and encouragement. Even the simplest of things: a warm wink of acknowledgment, a handshake with feeling. Their job description does not necessarily involve establishing an emotional bond, yet the patient in critical care is all about emotions: fear, doubt, humility, suffering, despair, isolation, desolation, angst . . .

Even today, I appreciate the fact that these amazing and talented people were often able to put themselves in my patient's ill-fitting, annoying, Dynarex nonskid unisex hospital sock slippers and that they didn't take for granted the crucial but often forgotten part of the modern Hippocratic oath that advises them to take seriously the "human" aspect of their commitment, to wit: "I will remember that there is art to medicine as well as science, and that warmth, sympathy, and understanding may outweigh the surgeon's knife or the chemist's drug."

As Larry David would say in his hilarious TV show *Curb Your Enthusiasm*, I am pret-ty, pret-ty, pret-ty, pret-ty lucky!

Minutes after Dael exits my room, Susan—my loving wife, Saviour, and constant visitor and pepper-upper—and I have an outrageous discussion with the nutritionist, whom we fondly call "The Gestapo Lady." *Follow the Rules to the Letter!* She is nothing less than a female Inspector Javert. I squirm as she tells us I can't eat this and I can't eat that and what I can't eat for the rest of my born days. (She happens to be right about grapefruit and sushi.)

I feel like giving this nurse the finger, yelling at her, and being unabashedly infantile, but instead, I choose to protest by quoting her the Delphic Oracle's two golden rules ("Nothing in excess, know thyself": remember these from the preceding chapter?) and explaining how, incredibly and inevitably, everything in life essentially boils down to these two wise ancient pieces of advice. She is giving me this funny look, after which I am hearing in my head the five eloquent words uttered by the great guitarist Chet Atkins: "Fight mediocrity tooth and nail."

Grrrrr.

Susan and I are still discussing the quandary of Rules vs. Flexibility, and how we are planning for me to eat in moderation Things Not Necessarily Good for My Heart but Good for My Psyche and My Soul. And we are reminiscing, fondly, about the story I have affectionately titled "Marie Pistorius and the Noshes."

It is the summer of 2004, and Susan and I are on the East Coast after our June Santa Barbara wedding. We have planned a trip to New York City (to visit friends and family), then on to my old summer camp in Maine, and finally to Williamstown, MA, to visit my alma mater.

Shortly after we arrive at the Williams campus, we find ourselves in the charming little home of George and Marie Pistorius. George, originally a Czech from Prague, was as kind and generous a man as you would ever want to meet. He was also a retired French professor, my mentor and thesis adviser when I was an undergrad, and, for the next five decades until his passing, a good and steadfast friend. Marie, a slight and shy woman, was every bit as sweet and kind as her husband.

After we chat and reminisce for a good while, it is time for the traditional sherry and noshes that hosting college professors and their wives are wont to serve up to their guests. George does the honors with the sherry, pouring Susan and me, then Marie and himself, nice full glasses of a prime Amontillado. (This word invariably evokes for me Poe's short story that includes this proper name.)

After we have enjoyed a few sips of sherry and lots of cheery small talk, Marie politely excuses herself from the living room and disappears into the kitchen. Three minutes later, she emerges, transporting a platter of Carr's English water crackers and a gorgeous wheel of oozy Brie. As she places them gently on the coffee table, I realize instantly that we have a problem.

"Marie," I begin timidly. "This is so thoughtful of you! I love Brie, but as you know, I've had some serious heart issues for a while now, and I really shouldn't—"

Without missing a beat, Marie apologizes sweetly in her heavy Czech accent: "Oh, I'm so sorry, I wasn't even thinking. Let me fetch you something else." And she disappears again into the bowels of the kitchen.

Three minutes later, she reemerges, this time holding a platter of Carr's English water crackers upon each of which sits a humongous *shmeer* of the finest French goose liver pâté. Susan and I look at each other and are laughing so hard inside that tears are streaming down our lungs.

Back at the hospital, for the next few weeks, I continue to have uncomfortably frequent encounters with my old friend, humility.

I am walking through the hallways of the fifth floor, hobbled and weak and holding onto my monitor and limping along like a goddam 105-year-old geezer.

I am witnessing, day by day, my deteriorating condition: my arms turning purple, my body losing weight rapidly, my legs becoming thinner and barely recognizable, my appetite for food and my passion for living waning by the hour.

I am lying helpless and half-naked on my bed watching attractive female nurses remove catheters from various body parts.

I am lying on a gurney in a cath lab waiting area, surrounded by mostly octogenarian patients who make me feel way older than I really am. I am staring out into space, feeling vulnerable and naked (in both senses), waiting to have a piece of kidney or liver or heart or lung snipped out of me, feeling like I am in a nightmare that refuses to end. Something cooked up by Poe or Kafka or Rod Serling. This wait sometimes lasts for two or three hours or more, during which time I am feeling neglected and abandoned by nurses and techs who are supposed to be telling me that my turn has come and wheeling me off to the lab. To pass the time, eyes closed, I am silently reciting the final stanza of W. H. Auden's poignant poem "Musée des Beaux Arts," which describes a painting by Peter Breughel the Elder and at the conclusion of which the mythical lad Icarus falls into the sea to his death (he has flown too close to the sun, and his wings of wax designed by his father, Daedalus, have melted), during which event no one even noticed the tragedy:

> *In Breughel's Icarus, for instance: how everything turns away*
> *Quite leisurely from the disaster; the ploughman may*
> *Have heard the splash, the forsaken cry,*
> *But for him it was not an important failure; the sun shone*
> *As it had to on the white legs disappearing into the green*
> *Water, and the expensive delicate ship that must have seen*
> *Something amazing, a boy falling out of the sky,*
> *Had somewhere to get to and sailed calmly on.*

After reciting these verses in my mind, I force myself, as always, to forbid these feelings of humility and helplessness and dependency and anonymity from discouraging or defeating me. The only person I will be with every second of my entire life, and on whom I can always depend, is myself. I must be strong and resilient and independent, even in these dire circumstances. When the existentialist writer Jean-Paul Sartre (in his play *Huis clos*, through his character Joseph) exclaimed, "Hell is other people," he was being, in my opinion, extreme and harsh and cynical. But I take his point.

Humility. From the Latin noun *humus*, or "ground." How perfect.

Still lying on the gurney, surrounded by misery and angst and preoccupied with my own pain and fears, I am contemplating, by association, another kind of humiliation, one of being brought down to Earth (or the ground), in this instance not a physical humbling, but an intellectual one. It has happened to me many times during my life, but two of these instances are rising to the surface of my consciousness right about now.

One freezing morning in December of 1990, I bump into Bert Sugar, the late great boxing guru, on the commuter train leaving Chappaqua, NY, where I then lived, and heading toward New York City, where I then worked in advertising. Bert and I often bumped into each other on the platform while awaiting the next train, and during the ride, we enjoyed kibitzing about sports and challenging each other with inanely esoteric trivia questions. But on this particular morning, it's the first time we have ever met. After I tell him I am a lifelong sports fanatic, we begin a nonstop conversation that ends an hour and change later, when the train arrives at Grand Central Station and we have to bid our fond adieus.

At one point during the ride, we begin to toss out trivia questions right and left at a dizzying speed. I am feeling mighty confident, because after the first few challenges, I am holding my own against him, despite the fact that his very advanced brain is a bottomless repository of sports data.

"Where was Willie Mays born?" Bert asks smugly.

"Fairfield, Alabama," I reply promptly, grinning inside.

"Which three Knicks players scored over thirty points in the game in which Wilt Chamberlain scored 100?" I query, arching my eyebrow defiantly.

"Richie Guerin, Willie Naulls, and Cleveland BUCKner," Bert ripostes, meticulously enunciating the initial syllable of the final name with a playfully vicious and supercilious snarl.

Game on.

After a few seconds of thought, I think I've got him. The perfect trivia question he'll never get immediately, if at all.

"Okay, which boxing champion had a last name that is a palindrome?" I ask cockily.

Now, this is a devilishly difficult question because it not only requires a thorough knowledge of boxing history—which Bert has in spades, and then some—but also 1. a knowledge of the meaning of the word *palindrome* (a word or phrase reading the same backward and forward; my personal favorite is "A slut nixes sex in Tulsa") and 2. the ability to make a speedy nexus between the word and the boxer.

In half a millisecond, without even blinking and as if he knew the answer before I even asked the question, Bert retorts, guns ablazing, "Willie PEP!" My spirit wilts under the heat of his broad, victorious grin.

The second instance of my being humbled by a brain nimbler than mine occurred in 1988, when I was working at the New York boutique ad agency Angotti Thomas Hedge. The creative assignment challenging me one Thursday morning is the result of a disturbingly vague strategy statement from my client: write a full-page print ad (copy only, no visuals) for the *New York Times* touting the quality of the steaks at the Smith & Wollensky steakhouse in New York City. Deadline: tomorrow.

After working for the entire morning and afternoon and beginning to feel the deadline pressure, I am attacked by a *furor poeticus*, and an idea (brilliant, in my humble opinion) just pops out—a gift from the gods—from somewhere inside my gray matter that I know is killer and that I know will save my creative ass. Aware of the fact that the best steaks in the world are considered to come from steer raised in a certain South American country, I am thinking that a strong yet tongue-in-cheek-modest concept based on this fact would fit the bill and be a powerful way to make the point. At the bottom of my layout is, simply, the Smith & Wollensky logo (a sketch of the restaurant and its name underneath). My copy, surrounded by white space:

SIX RESTAURANTS IN THE WORLD CAN PREPARE
  A PERFECT STEAK.
FIVE ARE IN ARGENTINA.

I stride into the office of Tom Thomas, the cofounder and executive creative director of the agency. Tom possesses a brilliant and agile mind for conceptual advertising and word-smithing and is a fair-minded and perspicacious critic. I plop my ad confidently on his desk and await, breath bated.

Tom reads the ad, flashes that subtle approving smile of his, then pauses thoughtfully before speaking. I can almost hear the wheels of his mind whirring feverishly.

"Great ad, Bob, really great" he says. Then another minute of thinking and glaring at the words. "But . . . shouldn't it be . . . *four*?"

At first, I am flummoxed, baffled, and bewildered (not to mention bewitched and bothered), until I realize what Tom means. And how brilliant his fix is. I should indeed have said:

SIX RESTAURANTS IN THE WORLD CAN PREPARE
A PERFECT STEAK.
FOUR ARE IN ARGENTINA.

This nuanced revision gives the restaurant a little wiggle room: instead of stating, mathematically, that it can prepare the only perfect steak in the US, or, for that matter, anywhere outside of Argentina, it implies that there may in fact be another steakhouse, somewhere out there on the planet, that can also prepare a perfect steak. A little wry modesty, but a statement that still oozes self-assurance and outrageously impressive product quality. The "revised" ad runs for decades, with great success, but whenever I see it or hear about it, I think not of my own writing ability, but rather, in all humility, of Tom Thomas's.

Now beginning my fourth hour of lying on the gurney and still awaiting the call and feeling mighty humbled, I continue to twiddle my cerebral thumbs and can't help thinking of probably my first real, adult experience with humility, this time not so much feeling intellectually inadequate, but rather feeling like a complete and total doofus.

It is the fall of 1963, and I am beginning my sophomore year of college. At this moment in time, my life is perfect. I am getting into the swing of everything: academics, sports, social life, earnest self-discovery. My days are filled with working hard (term papers, class discussions, preparing for exams) and playing hard (soccer practices, college mixers on the weekends, heated bridge games). And to top it all off, I am living in gorgeous Williamstown, MA, and it is early October and the autumn leaves are on fire and the sounds of the Beach Boys and the Chiffons and Sam Cooke and Del Shannon and Lesley Gore and the Four Seasons and Roy Orbison waft through the dorm and smells of fall and football and beer kegs and trees and flowers fill the sweet New England air.

Heaven.

And to top it all off, I have just purchased my first car ever, a British Racing Green MGB roadster, and I'm driving on one of those brilliant and wonderfully nippy New England Friday afternoons, the top down and the wind whipping through my hair, to Bennington College in Vermont (then restricted to women) to pick up a date and bring her back to Williams (then restricted to men) for the weekend. The drive from Williamstown to Bennington is about twenty minutes. I am so proud of my new car, and I am feeling so incredibly cool driving it. *I am the king of the world!*

I pick up my date, and we chat a while in my tiny new vehicle. I discover that she is not only gorgeous and hot, but she is also smart as a whip and funny. The whole, delicious enchilada.

On the way back to Williamstown, we chat some more, and I am feeling a real connection with my date, but just as important to me, I am thinking: *This is so cool, driving in my little MGB, here in heaven on Earth, free as a bird, feeling the wind and seeing the falling leaves—what could possibly be better than this?*

Driving on US-7 South, and as we get closer to campus, by dumb luck or fate or destiny or whatever you want to call it, and as if nothing could possibly make this afternoon more perfect, something happens that will in fact make this afternoon even perfecter: coming toward us and from the opposite direction is another MGB roadster, and a British Racing Green one, to boot. What are the chances of that happening on a first date? What makes this such an extraordinary opportunity to impress my date is that it is, of course, customary and part of the same-sports-car-etiquette thing either to flash your headlights or to wave nonchalantly at the person driving the same car and model as he or she is about to cross your path, so to speak.

My male adrenaline is out of control now, and I pounce into action. I am calm. I am cool. I am a human cucumber. I glance at my date, to see if she acknowledges the cool roadster etiquette that is about to take place. She smiles at me knowingly. I am feeling oh-so-suave and oh-so-debonnaire and oh-so-Don Juan. And now, the moment has arrived. I decide to go the cooler route of flicking on my headlights toggle switch. I reach for it and flick it on, all the while glancing at my date while sporting that smooth, stupid Fred Astaire grin. But because I am not yet that familiar with the dashboard, I must have flicked on the wrong switch, because instantly, the windshield wipers are activated. As my gorgeous date is laughing her gorgeous ass off, I smile feebly and offer some transparently fabricated jackass explanation to exculpate myself, like that's the way they do it in England; but inside, I am feeling like an utter nitwit and am dearly longing to crawl into the nearest hole and hide there until the end of time.

I am learning, admittedly with great difficulty, to accept all these insults that have rained upon my body and spirit while I am cooped up in the hospital, this humility, these humbling and vulnerable feelings and thoughts. After all, in the grand scheme of things and considering what's at stake, how important are what I look like and how much pain I am feeling? To combat these various insults and in order to mend my broken pride, I summon a series of flashbacks to my "fit" days. Competing in baseball, basketball, and squash. Playing semipro soccer in France. Being a teaching tennis pro in Tel Aviv, Paris, and Sonoma, CA. Playing pickup hoops at the age of fifty against a bunch of twentysomething college kids and rupturing my right Achilles (talk about humility!). Introducing rollerblading to the Israelis. Playing golf on five continents.

These memories fill me with renewed energy and the positive attitude of overcoming all my depression, doubts, fears, and dependency and the desire to return to the optimism of my old self. I think of the old "fight-or-flight" response: I am a fighter, not a flighter.

On the other hand, from where I'm sitting (or, rather, lying), it's hard to remain positive 24/7. Impossible, in fact. The half-full side of me is fighting really hard to be jolly, but the sheer mass of anxious thoughts, the arms that have become pincushions, the increasing bodily decrepitude, the uncertainty of ever getting a new heart, and the various nagging pains are constantly conspiring to depress the crap out of me. I am often able, by sheer force of will or a quick nap, to fend off this horde of gremlins. But not now.

So I'm lying in bed in my room, running out of patience and of time (as the survival clock ticks, my volatile pulmonary artery pressure and creatinine—kidney function—numbers aren't where my cardiologists want them to be for me to be put on the 1A waiting list), feeling lots of pain and general malaise, gaunt, underweight, and exhausted. I'm not at all in a good place. When, just in the nick of time and on cue, Susan is here for one of her frequent cheery visits. This time, she glides into my room, waltzing gracefully into my space like Loretta Young used to glide into her living room at the beginning of her eponymous 1950s TV show. Susan is a breath of fresh air replacing the stench of my negative thoughts, her beaming smile permeating the entire hospital room. She is holding in her right hand three large and festive helium balloons: a yellow Happy Face; a puppy that says, "I Love You"; and a big red one shaped, appropriately, like a heart. As the hours pass, even many days after she leaves them yoked to a chair, the balloons continue to float, carefree and buoyant and high above my bed, without descending, without deflating in a death spiral, gently bobbing symbols of love and life and hope.

Hope. The key to survival here, and the piece of driftwood I need in my ocean of negativity. I am pondering the idea that after releasing all the evils into the world when she opened her infamous box, Pandora finally closed it after they had all escaped, leaving only Elpis, or Hope, within. And I recite silently the opening stanza of an Emily Dickinson poem:

"Hope" is the thing with feathers—
That perches in the soul—
And sings the tune without the words—
And never stops—at all—

As my Balloons of Hope float above my bedside, O. Henry's short story "The Last Leaf" floats into my head. You know, the tale of Johnsy, the deathly sick young woman who has lost her desire to live as, one by one, the leaves of an ivy vine outside her bedroom window fall. In her misery, she is determined to die as soon as the last leaf falls, but in the nick of time, her life is saved when just before his own death, a neighbor, Old Behrman, a failed artist all his life, paints an ivy leaf on the outside of her window.

It is the masterpiece he had always wanted to achieve.

6

Big Yellow Taxi

Now I know how it feels to be doing time in San Quentin. To be waiting on death row, actually.

More tests. More biopsies to check for disease and infection: heart, liver, kidney, lung, bone marrow.

Bone marrow!

If I ever gave you one piece of advice based on my personal experience, it would be this: if you can avoid it, never, *ever* have a bone marrow biopsy! (The caveat: by all means feel free to have one, but *not* if you're on life-support IV drips that prevent you from having any kind of pain-numbing meds.)

In a nutshell, the procedure involves sticking a needle into an area around your hip, apparently for the sole purpose of precipitating the most excruciating pain that a human being can possibly feel without passing out. For me, the pain was so bad that I saw not only stars, but also constellations, meteors, meteoroids, asteroids, celestial bodies, comets, natural objects, planets, planetoids, planetesimals, quasars, moons, the Sun, galaxies, dwarf galaxies, satellites, nebulae, black holes, globular clusters, white dwarfs, and novas. Not to mention supernovas. And to make matters even worse, not only can you feel the pain, but you can actually *hear* it. (Just imagine adding a postproduction soundtrack to that old silent movie where the damsel in distress is tied down to a log and a buzz saw slowly approaches her skull.)

Adding insult to grave injury, before the procedure, one of the doctors tells me that the biopsy might feel "a bit uncomfortable." (I am trying to suppress my anger and laughter, simultaneously, as I write this.) I have always been puzzled by this peculiar use of euphemism by physicians. I know they're trying their very best to be comforting and to avoid putting any bad thoughts into your head, but come on, if there's ever been a time for honesty and brutal straightforwardness, this is it. Why don't they just tell you, "Now this is gonna hurt like a freaking sonuvabitch and will be excruciatingly unbearable, so be prepared, okay?" and get it over with? (For the record, my second favorite physician's euphemism is "Now, you might feel a little pinch," just before they shove a needle into your jugular vein while performing a heart biopsy.)

In fact, the pain I experienced during my bone marrow biopsy was so excruciating that I have officially placed it atop my personal list of the most physically painful moments I have ever endured during my lifetime.

And so, without further adieu—*ta-da!*—here's my Personal Top Ten Hit Parade of Physical Pain, from least to most agonizing:

10. Torn Achilles tendon

9. The slow, painstaking peeling off of surgical dress-
   ing with exceedingly sticky tape that has stuck to
   the hairs of my beard and neck, neglected during
   the shaving prep process before a heart biopsy—
   which involves sticking a needle into my right jugular vein and inserting first an introducer sheath and
   then a catheter, into which is threaded a very long
   wire with a tiny pair of forceps at the end that snips
   off three or four small pieces of heart tissue, all to
   check if there's any posttransplant cardiac rejection

8. Heart attack

7. Acute appendicitis

6. Sneezing during recovery from open-heart surgery,
   during which they cracked my breastbone and
   spread open my rib cage

5. Severe gout attack

4. Slowly pulling out an unthinkably long catheter
   from my penis in the shower, as instructed by my
   caring urologist over the phone, just after I had
   laser prostate surgery

3. Kidney (actually, uric acid) stones

2. Any pain whatsoever relating to my teeth

1. Bone marrow biopsy, hands down

More blood work. More Swan-Ganz catheters (stuck into
my neck and down to the right side of my heart, to measure
heart function, blood flow, and arterial pressures). More boredom. Monitors beeping day and night (I have not pulled an
all-nighter since college, and now am I pulling them galore).

Constant interruptions (vitals; blood draws; x-rays; cleaning women cleaning; consults with cardiologists and their fellows and residents, social workers, psychiatrists, and dietitians). More boredom. And, to be perfectly honest, a few of the nurses are real pains in the tush.

More tests to determine whether I am a perfect candidate for a transplant. The tough part about this is that some of my more important numbers (mainly pulmonary artery pressure and creatinine levels) always seem to fluctuate, diabolically, and until they settle down and reach the desired levels, my name will not be placed on the waiting list.

Days and weeks go by, tortoisely slow, and the light at the end of the tunnel seems decades away. I am not by nature a patient man, but I must force myself to be so. To retain my sanity, I often invoke (not always successfully, I must admit) the ancient Chinese aphorism: "Patience, and the mulberry leaf becomes a silk gown." And to retain my sense of humor, I often invoke the sardonic quip of Woody Allen: "Eternity is really long, especially towards the end."

But, of course, sanity doesn't always prevail in these circumstances. I mean, how can a person waiting to be put on the waiting list for a new heart and being sorely tested (with tests) and being interrupted every eleven minutes possibly be patient? Especially if that patient is *me*?

In my hospital bed (where else?), I am reflecting on the cruel irony of the word *patient*. Like the word *passion*, it derives from the Latin (*pati*) and Greek (*pathein*) words that mean "to suffer." At its core, then, being patient means to suffer, as does being *a* patient. As a human being, personally, I am always patient (one who suffers) when it comes to writing or doing anything I love that is difficult, because I adore the process—and the passion—and know the ultimate rewards and what is necessary and required to reap them. But in general, impatience happens to be one of the most egregious of my many flaws and has been ever since I can remember. As a kid, I was always impatient when I took tests at school, propelled by my desire to finish first. I always wanted to do my very best, of course, but somehow, speed was my strongest motivation, fueled by a combination of adrenaline, metabolism, and competition. And—it seems silly now at my age, when I savor my every bite—the same velocity and impatience applied when it came to the dining room table, where I always drove myself to finish first. Except when Mom served up the odious combo of salmon croquettes and succotash, which I ate at a moss-growing pace before finally negotiating with her to have just one more bite before arriving, at last, at the agreed-upon not-quite-finish line.

But being (a) patient in a hospital is quite another story; and now, sorely tested by the endless waiting to be eligible for a new heart, it takes center stage. In fact, it is making me ponder one of the "paradoxes" of the Greek philosopher Zeno of Elea called "Achilles and the Tortoise." This conceit "proves" the *illusion* of motion (clearly an absurd thought), by demonstrating that Achilles (a hero of the Trojan War who, when he ran, could probably make Usain Bolt appear snail-like), in a race with a tortoise, could never pass the lethargic reptile, because he first had to reach the spot where the tortoise was when Achilles began to run, by which time the tortoise would have itself advanced forward. And so on and so on, for each segment of the race. This is called a reductio ad absurdum. Similarly, in my bed at Cedars-Sinai, I am getting the feeling that somehow, I can never "catch up" with my potential new heart, that no matter how long and patiently I wait to qualify for it, something will go wrong, or delays will beget delays, and it will elusively slither ahead, always out of my reach.

But hey, ya never know, and sometimes patience pays off. Susan and I are told the good news: I have at long, long last been put on the 1A list for a heart transplant! (Yes, Virginia . . .)

This is actually *great* news, since 1. many hospitals don't perform transplants on patients over sixty-five, much less on those over seventy, but Cedars-Sinai is one of the few places that even consider patients over seventy and 2. most often, a recipient has to wait many, many months and sometimes even years to receive a new heart (and in a frighteningly significant number of cases, potential recipients die waiting for a new heart—and specifically, about one in five patients with end-stage heart disease die within ninety days). In my case, being put on the 1A list was due to a combination of factors: I have type B blood, which means that I can receive a heart from a donor who has either type B or type O (the universal donor) and also that the waiting list for type B patients is shorter than it is for the more common type O patients (since the latter can only receive hearts from type O donors); my heart is in horrible shape, which means that I am in urgent need of a new one; my body is in good shape aside from the cardiac issues, which means that for my age, I have a better chance to survive the long surgery and tolerate a new heart inside me; and I have unbelievably strong (and deeply appreciated) support from my cardiology team at Cedars-Sinai on the

Committee That Decides Your Fate (which also includes the incredibly supportive cardiologist Ajay Srivastava from Scripps La Jolla), maybe because we all get along so well and maybe because they consider Susan as the perfect person who will take great and loving care of me when I am recuperating and maybe because they somehow see in me someone who—aside from meeting the criteria listed above—is worth saving. Which means everything to me.

The bad news: the wait—now for a new heart—seems endless once again.

More days creep by, and I am flooded—against my will or because of it?—by a horrendous thought, a thought of unimaginable perversion and grotesquerie. I am almost ashamed to say it, but I am actually hoping with all my cardiac organ that someone out there will accidentally perish in a car or motorcycle crash—and ASAP, I might add—in order to save my life. Bad things do inevitably happen, after all. This thought, as horrific and ethically abhorrent as it might sound, is, paradoxically, totally justified: in this situation, how could I possibly blame myself, or be blamed, for self-interest and the desire to survive, for both me and my family and friends?

Looking out my window one sunny morning, I am feeling imprisoned. Isolated. Segregated. A pariah. Like some criminal, or a leper in a colony. Like Quasimodo and Frankenstein. Like van Gogh and Beethoven. Like Camus's Meursault and Kafka's Gregor Samsa. I am, to paraphrase the wry 1950s comedian George Gobel, feeling like the world is a tuxedo and I'm a pair of brown shoes. The ironic paradox is that I do belong here because of obvious reasons, but the ordeal of being in here makes me feel like escaping, like being out there. My contradictory feelings of gratitude for being in here and anguish at not being out there are a continual frustration and challenge. And the only way I can deal with them (I can't sleep, and I don't want to ignore or deny them) is to ponder. My favorite escape mechanism, but at the same time my way of trying to resolve problems. And, just as important, thinking is one of my passions, and now it's a way to comfort myself and to give myself a feeling of peace amidst all this turmoil.

Still looking out the window, I am pondering further the concepts of dichotomy, paradox, contradiction, and conflict—all frustrating yet essential components of the human condition.

Syzygy is perhaps my favorite of the some half-million to one million words (depending on your source) in the English language, just nudging ahead of *chthonic*. Not only because of its odd spelling, but mostly because it can denote, alternatively and simultaneously, two things that are contradictory, both a conjunction and an opposition. The word is not used very frequently (surprise!), except in astronomy, to describe, for example, solar and lunar eclipses or a new moon (the sun and moon are in conjunction) and a full moon (the sun and moon are in opposition). But I like it anyway, because it makes me think of the contradictory yet complementary nature of many of life's important issues, especially those that are being evoked in me by what I have endured so far during my hospital stay.

Imprisonment and freedom, for example. And how much I hate being cooped up in here, but at the same time, this cooping makes me realize how much more I can (and will, assuming I get out of here alive) appreciate the simple freedom of being out there. This makes me reflect on how everything seems to exist only in relation to its opposite. There would be no life without death, and vice versa. There would be no absence without presence, and vice versa. I would not be so bored here if I were not, by contrast, habitually busy, productive, and passionate about my life. It is an ancient concept, really, going back at least to Plato's Opposites Argument in his dialogue *Phaedo*.

All of which brings to my mind the fascinating concept of *ullage*. I love this word, too, because it means absolutely nothing. *Literally!* It refers to the empty portion of a cask or a bottle of wine or a glass. And the beauty of this concept is that you can't have full without empty, and vice versa. What a perfect metaphor: each side of the equation can only define itself in relation to its opposite! The only exception, of course, is the wonderful scene in the film classic *The Bishop's Wife*, in which the angel Dudley (the wonderful Cary Grant) keeps refilling the wine glass magically with a flick of his finger, to the utter surprise of Professor Wutheridge (the wonderful Monty Woolley) each time he attempts to take a sip.

Actually and paradoxically, now that I am thinking about it here in my hospital room, every single meaningful value I have ever espoused has an equally viable value attached to its opposite. I see these pairs, these dichotomies, not as positive vs. negative, as is often the perception, but as being in a very deep sense symbiotic, both contradictory and complementary. Whether it's success and failure, passion and struggle, justice and injustice, luck and self-determination, humility and hubris, knowing and not knowing, or imprisonment and freedom, the apparent antagonists are always symbiotic, joined at the hip with their opposite number, like a plover bird cleaning a crocodile's teeth.

A few days later, I am ruminating once again on what it's like to be trapped in a hospital and divorced from the outside world. What it's like to have things taken away that you're used to having: freedom, self-esteem, pride, sense of community, relationships. How you don't know what you've got till it's—

Suddenly, the Joni Mitchell (no relation) song "Big Yellow Taxi" leaps into my brain:

> *Don't it always seem to go*
> *That you don't know what you've got till it's gone?*

I spend the next few hours appreciating many of the good things in my life, now that they have been (temporarily, I hope) stolen from me.

Here, in fact, in my little room on the fifth floor at Cedars-Sinai Medical Center in Los Angeles, California, music has saved my life, not literally, but pretty damn close. Joni's words have inspired me to find the energy (and at the urging of Susan, who loves music just as much as I do) to open up my laptop and listen to some of my favorites on my iTunes: James Taylor, Joe Cocker, Randy Newman, Elton John, Phil Collins, John Fogerty, Leon Redbone, Francesco De Gregori, Georges Brassens, Leo Kottke, Chet Atkins, The Beatles, Keb' Mo', Dixie Chicks, Beethoven, Mozart, Brahms, Handel, George Gershwin, The Platters, Gilbert & Sullivan, Ella Fitzgerald, Seals & Crofts, Christine McVie, Dan Fogelberg, Jacques

Brel, Van Morrison, Bruce Springsteen, Roberto Vecchioni, Indigo Girls, Ramblin' Jack Elliott, Jackson Browne, Zac Brown Band . . .

It's amazing how music can transport you away from the reality of the moment. Uplift your spirits and move you and calm your nerves and energize your senses and placate your soul. As William Congreve said in *The Mourning Bride*, "Music hath charms to soothe a savage breast." And by now, after spending lo these many months cooped up in hospitals, my breast is plenty savage.

My mind flashes back to all the musical highlights of my life so far and how much they have enriched my existence: listening to all the operettas of Gilbert and Sullivan and early rock 'n' roll as a kid; waiting in college for the next explosively revolutionary Beatles LP to be released; playing my acoustic guitars (Martins and Guilds); giving folk concerts in France; thousands of hours of pleasure listening to artists from Abba to Zac Brown Band; and attending awesome concerts given by performers like Leon Russell, Ramblin' Jack Elliott, Leon Redbone, Odetta, Leo Kottke, Elton John, Paul Simon, Taj Mahal, Karla Bonoff, Bob Dylan, James Taylor, Livingston Taylor, Tom Rush, and Randy Newman.

Now don't get me wrong: I happen to love the other arts—literature and painting and the plastic arts and architecture and dance and theater and film and the culinary arts and photography and mime. But for me, music is even more immediate and more sensual. And life-saving, especially when you're really sick and running out of time and patience.

Days continue to creep by, with the same old cast of characters: yet more X-rays, Swan-Ganz catheters, ultrasounds, waiting, boredom, biopsies, and extreme physical and mental trauma. The good news: despite my still-fluctuating numbers (notably, as ever, creatinine and pulmonary artery pressure), I am still on the transplant waiting list. The bad news: I am still on the transplant waiting list.

One fine morning, a very nice RN enters my room and performs the perfunctory tasks: taking vitals (blood pressure, temperature, oxygen level, and pulse rate), drawing blood, testing arterial pressure, removing and cleaning dressings from my arms and neck, giving me more warm blankets, measuring my urine output. And we chat.

"How you feeling?" the nurse asks me a tad perfunctorily.

"Oh, not too bad," I reply semiunenthusiastically, transparently revealing my pain and discouragement. Then, unable to come up with something witty or original or even meaningful, for some unknown reason I resort to a lame line from a comic book I had read about sixty years ago: "Actually, I feel like a million bucks—green and wrinkled."

She emits a forced yet charitable smile.

"Y'know," she says apologetically, "If I would've known you were feeling so bad, I would've been a little gentler with you when I was removing your dressings."

Now, I am extremely appreciative of the good-natured nature of her response. In fact, I smile back at her accordingly. But inside of me, I am frowning and disapproving and wagging my right index finger at her and awakened from my mental torpor. As it happens, the phrasing "If I would have . . . I would have . . ." (instead of the correct "If I had . . . I would have . . .") is way up there, just nudging ahead of "irregardless," on my Top Ten List of Pet Grammatical Peeves.

For a split second, I am debating whether or not to correct her grammar. Will I offend her, or will I do her a favor by shining on her the bright light of the Proper Use of Our Rich and Nuanced Native Language? I conclude that if she is offended, she is either paranoid or terribly insecure, and that's on her, so—delicately and, as always, with beneficence aforethought—I make the needed correction.

She takes kindly to my didactic comment. When appropriate, I feel obliged to point out this type of error as a "Good Grammar Samaritan," because I believe that language usage reflects on you personally. (I did it with my kids and my students, and sometimes, as now, with perfect strangers!) And I myself am always eager to learn new things, from any source, whether human or mechanical. But now, I am sort of regretting my correction: Frankly, who cares? And I put it in perspective: So you make a mistake? I'm on life support, hanging on by a thread, waiting for a new heart, so how much could or should it matter?

If I would've known how unimportant this was right now, I would've not let it bother me.

All this is evoking memories of my graduate days at Harvard. It was, and still is, a pretty "brainy" environment, and I found it quite stimulating and challenging. On the other hand, I always felt a bit out of place in the halls of academe, because part of me is not really an intellectual, but, rather, is athletic and down-to-earth and doesn't take itself too seriously. It is this schizophrenic frame of mind (am I an intellectual snob or just a regular guy who likes to be grammatically helpful?) that is bringing to my mind the following—apocryphal—story.

One crisp fall day, a young, innocent freshman is walking across Harvard Yard on the Cambridge campus. He is in awe of the environment and has a proud, beaming look on his face, and why not? He happens to be the very first student from the state of Idaho to have been accepted as a Harvard undergraduate on a full scholarship.

But he seems to be a bit disoriented and needs assistance. As luck would have it, directly opposite him and strolling in his direction is a crusty-looking, mustachioed, silver-haired, nattily dressed professor bedecked in a deerstalker (Sherlock Holmes) cap, a blue Oxford button-down shirt with embroidered initials on the cuffs, a perfectly positioned crimson tie with little white birds soaring on its surface, perfectly pressed charcoal-gray slacks, an olive sports jacket with tan suede elbow patches, and an exceedingly buffed pair of cordovan wingtips.

"Excuse me, Sir, but could you please tell me where the library's at?" the freshman from the Gem State inquires.

"Why, young man, are you not aware of the fact that you must *never* end a sentence with a preposition?" the professor ripostes haughtily.

"Oh, excuse me, Sir," the young man says after hesitating a moment, "but could you please tell me where the library's at, *asshole*?"

Speaking of the academic/regular guy conflict in my mind, I am suddenly recollecting a scene that took place during one of our trips to Italy to visit Giuseppe and Maria. Susan and I and our two dear Roman friends are driving around Umbria, and we stop in Assisi to see the town, including Giotto's cycle of twenty-eight frescoes, "The Legend of Saint Francis," in the upper church of the Basilica di San Francesco.

We somehow end up separating into two groups, Maria and I and then Giuseppe and Susan. As Maria and I walk past each of the late-thirteenth-century frescoes (I had first studied Giotto in 1962, in my Art 101 course at Williams), she reads to me from an Italian guidebook the punctilious and excruciatingly long-winded details of each fresco (date, origin, source, technique, description of the action, and so on). I find the descriptions fascinating, although after a while, a part of me—the impatient, nonacademic side—is screaming frantically to be released from the tedium. We take twenty-five minutes to complete her guided tour, and by the end, I feel both edified and fit to be tied.

At that point, we meet up with Susan and Giuseppe, who had completed their own tour in a little under six minutes and had been chatting for the past nineteen.

"So, how was the tour?" Susan asks.

"Amazing!" I reply, arching my right eyebrow.

"Ah," Susan says, totally getting my gesture.

"Yeah, it was really educational and detailed and, well—"

"*Noioso!* " Maria says, a sweetly candid smile filling her cherubic face.

"She said, 'boring!'" I tell Susan, who generally understands Italian pretty well. We are all in hysterics. But that's not the best part.

"And how'd *your* guided tour go?" I ask Susan.

"Great!" Susan says. "Giuseppe told me, as we walked by the frescoes, 'Saint Francis. He was born . . . he lived . . . he died.'"

The four of us are now cracking up uncontrollably, tears racing down our eight cheeks. And through my hysteria and my tears, the academic and the iconoclastic regular guy in me are both having a good ol' time.

Back here in Cedars-Sinai, the past few days have been especially rough: my creatinine level is, as is often the case, too high (vacillating between 2.5 and 4, but the docs want it to be below 2); I am on the 1A list, then off it, then on the cusp, then on it again; now, after biopsies, they find a suspicious something on my right lung, then one in my right kidney; I am exhibiting high blood sugar levels, water retention (I am being given large doses of IV diuretics), physical weakness, and shaking of hands and legs from all the prednisone; and—worst of all perhaps—mental feebleness has somehow crept in: I am having serious trouble for the first time with the Sunday *New York Times* crosswords.

And let's not for a moment forget the indigestible food. This may sound a bit harsh, because on the other hand, the dietary staff definitely deserves loads of credit for cooking three squares a day for many hundreds of patients, and they are certainly constrained to follow strict bureaucratic culinary guidelines. But let's face it: it's not likely that too many of the cooking staff has ever won (or will ever win, for that matter) a James Beard Award. Without going into details about their odorless, tasteless, hard-to-cut, hard-to-swallow, bland, repetitive, lukewarm offerings, I will simply say that for the past week or so, I have been reduced, by process of utter elimination, to three meals a day, each one consisting of a bottle of rich chocolate Boost and a board of stale matzoh (as redundant as that may sound) topped with a *shmeer* of semitasteless peanut butter.

Susan is my Saviour once again, though, smuggling in illegal merchandise behind the backs of the ubiquitous and ever-vigilant nurses: bags of Skinny Pop popcorn and Tate's chocolate chip cookies, slices of watermelon, breaded chicken cutlets, her world-renowned meatballs and angel hair pasta . . . How I appreciate her efforts, not only her food smuggling, but also her commuting every day for two to four hours, depending on traffic patterns and starting point—from our home in Carlsbad or her daughter's (and our new twin granddaughters') in Agoura or her sister's in Santa Monica—and especially negotiating the brutal LA traffic! And her giving up the creation of her wonderful art for who-knows-how-long. And her worrying about me, and being with me. And her optimism. And her nurturing love.

My endless days are lightened up not only by Susan's visits, but also by those of two physicians who are on the case but aren't obliged to see me daily. The amazing thing is, though, that they do!

Larry Froch is a friendly, warm, bright, down-to-earth nephrologist who checks in on me every day, not only to examine me and see that my kidney is (so to speak) keeping itself above water, but also to shmooz. We talk about a great many things, medical and otherwise, and he never fails to lift up my spirits. One day he even brings in his precocious teenage son, and the three of us chat about his science project and his plans for the future.

Michael Levine is a friendly, warm, bright, down-to-earth pulmonologist who checks in on me every day, not only to examine me and (so to speak) clear the air about the condition of my lungs, but also to shmooz. He is an iconoclast, which I find appealing, because I am one, too. Whenever I mention how rigid and numbingly unbending the hospital rules are, he is constantly reminding me that you gotta play the game to get what you want (a new heart), that you gotta put up with all the crap and all the orders and be nice to everyone (I am in fact constantly being evaluated for my attitude, comportment, cooperation, and mental stability, on pain of being ripped off the heart transplant waiting list). He is right, of course, but it's nice to know that he and I share the same spirit of rebelliousness. Once, after a passionate discussion about "the powers that be," I quote to him something that Mr. Bumble in Dickens's *Oliver Twist* said: ". . . the law is a ass—a idiot." Michael laughs, and before he leaves, we execute a spirited fist bump, the ritual ending to each of our visits.

One steamy afternoon, I am once again staring out my window, which continues to be a double-edged metaphor, at once the very embodiment of my access to the outside world and at the same time the very symbol of my imprisonment behind it.

I am thinking at this moment about freedom, about getting the hell outta here and enjoying the open air and the open skies and the open world (after, hopefully, my open-heart surgery).

I am meditating on the time in my life on Earth when I was freest of all encumbrances, obligations, rules and regulations, and tethers (whether parental, academic, or professional).

It is August of 1966, nearly fifty years ago. I have just received my college degree (a BA in French), and I am sailing to France on a then-thirty-year-old freighter named *Aurelia* to spend a year teaching English in Angers on a Fulbright Fellowship, along with fifty-odd other fellowship recipients who will be stationed in other Gallic destinations. It is the first time in my life that I am in an environment pretty much devoid of structure of any kind. I am free as a seagull. My belongings include a duffel bag stuffed with clothes and a few books, a Martin 0018 acoustic guitar, and a bulky (primitive by today's standards) reel-to-reel Grundig tape recorder and four BASF tapes that contain about a million or so songs (Joan Baez, The Beatles, PP&M, Mississippi John Hurt, Leadbelly, Dave Van Ronk . . .).

I am not only free of writing term papers and taking exams and writing a senior thesis and going to fellowship interviews (although I still to this day cherish my college experience), but I will also be liberated, for the entire coming year, from most "traditional" restrictions: other than showing up to teach my classes, I will have no other pedagogical duties or schedules, I will take no orders (or guff) from anyone, I will be allowed to make up my own syllabi and course plans and to come and go as I please to and from the lycée (the Lycée de Garçons David d'Angers) I've been assigned to (uh-oh: I hope that crusty preposition-at-the-end-of-sentences-obsessed Harvard prof doesn't come after me!), I will be free to go anywhere I want on the frequent recesses and vacations (I end up traveling to Brittany, Paris, Morocco, London, Surrey, Belgium, the Netherlands, and the *Schwarzwald* in Germany). I have scrawled my John Hancock, in my brain, on a Mental and Physical Declaration of Independence, and I will devote my coming year to the passionate pursuit of Life, Liberty, and the pursuit of Happiness.

All I remember from the journey is that it took us ten days to sail from New York to Le Havre, that *Aurelia* didn't have stabilizers (so the passage had its rough spots), and that I spent all of my time drinking, dancing, reading, making out, and making out my lesson plans. Especially memorable was drinking and dancing into the wee hours to the sounds emanating from the jukebox, the most memorable of which was the Cuban song "Guantanamera," played incessantly, sung by the Sandpipers, and arranged by Pete Seeger. I can still hear the chorus to this very day.

Guantanamera, guajira Guantanamera . . .

Back to my hospital window. I am at heart an optimist and a fighter, but at this moment, I am filled with a paralyzing sadness. The feelings of inactivity and being cooped up are really, really getting to me and are evoking inside of me, in my cerebral mirror, the image of a sad, mangy dog imprisoned in a pound: the forlorn look, the empty gaze, the beaten-down mien. My alter ego, Fido, just sitting there with his doggy thoughts.

Just waiting to grab someone's heart.

I am watching people way down there on the ground walking, meeting, talking, eating, gesticulating, arguing, embracing, texting, hoping, planning, carrying on with their lives. And I am picturing the world without me.

Will my demise simply mean that there will be one less person in the US (319 million, as opposed to 319,000,001)? And one less person in the world (7.4 billion, as opposed to 7,400,000,001)? I do not particularly believe in the concept of legacy, in my leaving some sort of meaningful footprint after my demise. But, I am still thinking: *What has my life added up to?* To borrow from Jean Valjean, in the theatrical version of Victor Hugo's epic novel *Les Misérables*, I am now asking myself, "Who Am I?" Who are *all of us* in the universe?

And yet: I have a wife and kids and family and friends who love me, I have achieved a few things of some value in my life, I have given pleasure to a bunch of people. *Doesn't this count?*

I am remembering Linda Loman's poignant and pathetic monologue in Act I of Arthur Miller's glorious play *Death of a Salesman*. About her mediocre, unsuccessful husband, Willy, she tells her son Biff, "He's not to be allowed to fall in his grave like an old dog. Attention, attention must finally be paid to such a person."

The world *without* me?

But then, I am thinking of all my recent, human feelings of self-doubt, frustration, failure, insufficiency, fragility, vulnerability, and humility. And of that scene on the bridge between the flawed George Bailey and Bert the cop toward the end of the film *It's a Wonderful Life*, when George ultimately realizes that he did, after all, make a real, palpable difference in other people's lives.

The world *with* me!

7
Wounded Deer

When I was twelve, I tacked onto my bulletin board a sign with an anonymous quote written on it. The words, which amused me no end then and which have remained locked inside my brain for six decades, read, "One day while I sat musing, sad and lonely and without a friend, a voice came to me from out of the gloom, saying 'Cheer up, things could be worse.' So I cheered up . . . and sure enough things got worse."

This happens to me sometimes. Like *now*.

Susan and I are told the devastating news: during one of my many scans to determine whether I am a perfect heart recipient, they found a largish mass in my right kidney. And they did a biopsy. And now they are telling us that the tumor is, as feared, malignant (renal cell carcinoma, to be precise) and I will need to be removed from the heart transplant list indefinitely and to undergo surgery (a partial nephrectomy) ASAP to remove a little less than half of my kidney and they hope my old, sick heart can tolerate and survive the trauma of the surgery and depending on the results, my fate will be sealed: either it is too late and the cancer has spread and a transplant will be out of the question and there's no hope, or they got it all and it hasn't spread and I will be put back on the waiting list and then who knows?

Sheesh.

First the sick heart and the waiting for a new one, and now the sick kidney and the waiting for the surgery and the results. Life has first thrown me a curveball, and now it is delivering a spitball with saliva oozing all over the seams.

After Susan leaves my room, I am lying on my bed and staring up at the ceiling. I am alone and filled with a feeling that makes terror look pale and weak and inconsequential by comparison. I am missing Susan and I am missing my health and I am missing my kids and I am missing my friends and I am missing my life. For the moment, a fake smile on my face, I find myself in the uncomfortable and unfamiliar role of the tragic clown Pagliaccio (you know, the guy with the fake smile to mask *his* broken heart).

Which compels me to recall an evening I spent in Paris in 1959, the first time I ever saw the iconic French mime Marcel Marceau perform in person. He is portraying his persona Bip the Clown in a hilarious skit called "The Mask Maker." At one point, after affixing on his face, alternately, a smiling mask and a frowning mask, the mask maker puts on the one with a huge smile (the mask of comedy?) and then, suddenly and for no apparent reason, is unable to remove it from his face. It is stuck, and the cherubic grin is frozen on the mask maker's face. Try as he might to remove the mask (with his bare hands and an imaginary chisel and hammer), he can't. And, the smile still pasted on his face, the mask maker paces, is furious and despairing and frustrated, throws his arms up in the air in disgust, begs in a why-me? pose, sighs and curses silently.

On a deeper level, I am now relating to the natural reaction to despair by protecting myself and putting on a (fake) smile. It is all very sad. And very funny.

Easier said than done, this aphorism about looking at the bright side. Right now, I am in shock about the cancer news. I am trying as hard as I can to be sunny, to focus in my head on the Peggy Lee song (with Benny Goodman on clarinet) "On the Sunny Side of the Street":

> *Grab your coat, get your hat*
> *Leave your worries on the doorstep*
> *Just direct your feet*
> *To the sunny side of the street.*

Trouble is, I have no coat or hat, there is no doorstep, and there is no sun or street—literally and figuratively—here in the hospital.

I am ruminating on the concept of cancer. *I have cancer? Who, me?* I keep repeating to myself in disbelief. *Huh?* No family history, no warning signs, just out of the blue? As the reality that my body has indeed been attacked by this grave affliction begins to calcify, I am thinking of the friends I have lost to this scourge, including dear friends from summer camp, high school, college, and beyond. And of Susan's Mom, Lila, who died far too young at the age of 67, whom I never had the pleasure of meeting (she died seven years before I met Susan), and who was an essential part of my wife's life. Not to mention the many millions of people who have died of this horrible affliction, and the anguish of their spouses and partners and parents and children and relatives and friends and colleagues and acquaintances. It's almost too much to digest right now.

I am recollecting—with pride and pleasure—a public service TV commercial about breast cancer that I wrote and produced in Tel Aviv for the Gitam ad agency, in 1994. Before I was commissioned to do it, the Israeli government had done a spot using a "talking head," a well-known actress who, speaking to the camera, implored women to give themselves regular breast self-examinations. But now they wanted something stronger, more immediate, more urgent. The concept I came up with was quite simple, actually. No talking heads, no actors, no spiel. After doing hours of research in the main library in Tel Aviv, I compiled a series of twenty or so works of art—by painters like Raphael, Botticelli, and Modigliani—depicting various women in stylized poses placing a finger (or two) or a hand on one of their breasts. I created a montage of these portraits, one softly dissolving into another and each in a different position on the screen. No voiceover, just the succession of images, with the dramatic opening of Beethoven's Symphony #3 mixed in the background. At the very end of the spot, a female voiceover simply asks women to do regular breast self-examinations. The result reflected the incredible power of art to deliver a message on a very moving, personal level.

How ironic that now it is *I* who have been attacked by the dreaded disease!

In the midst of my glumness, I begin to sing silently the hilarious lyrics to "Always Look on the Bright Side of Life," as sung by Graham Chapman, Eric Idle, and all the other crucifixion victims in the final scene of the movie *Monty Python's Life of Brian.* I can't resist smiling broadly, even though I am feeling much closer now to Pagliaccio and Bip the Clown than to anything approaching cheerful.

Meanwhile, I'm losing weight like crazy. Thirty-five pounds, to be exact, which doesn't sound all that horrific except for the fact that it represents 23.3 percent of my original total body weight before I became sick. In my bed, I am staring at my body and all its new flaws. I am thinking of the upcoming surgery and the subsequent awaiting of my fate. Nothing is ever easy in life, and it's all about The Struggle.

And The Fear.

As I am enduring my process and dealing with my struggle, the refrain of a song wafts into my brain, a simple yet haunting song of great beauty and consequence, and with a deeply meaningful and appropriate message for me. It will waft up there many more times while I am here. The song is "La leva calcistica della classe '68" ("Soccer Draft, Class of '68"), a gorgeous paean to the courage and spirit of youth written and sung by my very favorite Italian *cantautore* (singer-songwriter), the amazing Francesco De Gregori. The beginning of the refrain, which expresses the mentality of the brave protagonist, a twelve-year-old soccer player by the name of Nino, comes into focus now:

Ma Nino non aver paura di sbagliare un calcio di rigore . . .

These elegantly simple and inspiring eleven words (ten in English: "But Nino is not afraid of missing a penalty kick . . .") stop me in my bedridden tracks.

I have taken many crucial penalty kicks in my own soccer career, so I know full well what these words mean. The game is on the line, and nobody is there in the penalty area except you and the opposing goalkeeper. The pressure is palpable, and you have only two choices: *fear or courage.* Period. You can doubt yourself and be afraid of missing and of disappointing your teammates and your coach . . . or you can have inner strength, confidence, and a plan. Half empty or half full, the ball is in your pitch.

As ever, I am thinking, as I hum De Gregori's lyrics silently, of sports as a metaphor for life. And how, in both spheres . . . *fear paralyzes!* And how, in both spheres, of all the powerful negative thoughts imaginable, fear is right up there at the top of the list.

I am visualizing the scene in the song with me (substituting for Nino) preparing to take the penalty kick, and the two scenarios: Am I going to blow it and lose the game? Or . . . I'm gonna nail this baby: I'll feint left and, using deception of body and eyes, go top right corner. Me against the keeper, and I will outfox him, no question. No negative thoughts, just desire and determination. For me, the choice is a no-brainer: *I shall not allow fear to defeat me.*

And now, as I hum the Italian lyrics and lie here in my hospital bed, the sports-as-life metaphor is in full bloom and I am Nino and Nino is I and the goalkeeper—he alone standing between me and triumph— is Death.

And I'll be damned if Death is gonna beat me!

I am contemplating this concept intensely, this quandary that has fascinated me my whole adult life. How all good things come as the result of struggle. I am thinking of the Greek tragedian Aeschylus's mellifluous *"Pathema, mathema,"* "Lessons through suffering." Which leads me naturally to the Latin aphorism *"Per aspera ad astra,"* "To the stars through hardships," which I learned at my high school, Poly Prep in Brooklyn, in Mr. Winder's eighth-grade Latin class. At that time, at age thirteen, I viewed the phrase as a lovely clump of accusatives, alliteration, and consonance, fodder for the brain and not the heart, as I had not yet experienced any significant loss, setback, failure, excruciating challenge, or cataclysm in my life.

Little did I know.

In fact, I was asked—and was deeply honored—to give the commencement address at my high school alma mater in 2007. And one of the main motifs throughout the speech was this very concept of *per aspera ad astra*. Imagine: I was talking to these fine young students, not about going out into the world and doing good and their future is bright and their whole lives are ahead of them and how happy and successful they will be and how important a good education is. No, there I was, behind a pulpit and facing all the graduates and their parents and relatives and friends and teachers, talking to them about the importance of failure and struggle!

I told them, as I tell myself constantly, that dreams and achievement and success are worthless without hard work and struggle. As UCLA basketball coaching legend John Wooden aptly opined, "Nothing will work unless you do." I told them that this is true in work, play, love, marriage, raising children, community service, whatever. And that without this counterpoint of struggle and challenges, passion is oddly incomplete.

Ullage, anyone?

In the end, nothing excellent or worthwhile is easy, and those who make it "seem easy"—whether they are athletes, actors, singers, musicians, composers, writers, artists, architects, educators, doctors, designers, lawyers, carpenters, firefighters, florists, nurses, mimes, chefs, accountants, realtors, philosophers, interior designers, film directors, programmers, scientists, dentists, translators, pilots, librarians, interpreters, engineers, pharmacists, or therapists—have in fact really struggled and studied and worked their butts off to perfect their disciplines and to arrive at that high level of proficiency. There is a wonderful Italian word, coined by Castiglione in his *The Book of the Courtier*, that expresses this concept. The word is *sprezzatura*. (To see *sprezzatura* in action, all you have to do is watch the "Sunday Jumps" scene in the old 1951 film *Royal Wedding* where Fred Astaire dances with the hat rack.)

As I await my nephrectomy surgery and my fate, lying here anxiously in bed, I am thinking about how I must not just endure the struggle, the process, but actually *embrace* it. I am remembering what the great French poet Paul Valéry said of this unending process (in this case, regarding writing): "*On ne termine jamais un poème, on l'abandonne*," "You never finish a poem, you abandon it." Writing, as Valéry well knew, is an excruciating, ever-evolving *process* (etymologically, this word means "going forward") that only ends when another project must be begun or when a deadline arrives. Being a writer, of course, I know this all too well. There you are, sometimes from 8 a.m. until 2 a.m. the next day, in front of your blank computer screen or empty writing pad, the white (or yellow) page beckoning like a Siren. Sometimes in the wee hours, asleep, searching in your subconscious for just the right word, the right nuance, you awake in a cold sweat with just the word you have been searching for all those hours and days! Agony? Well, yes, but if you are a serious writer, you must love it and know that every time, you will savor the process and fight through the sleeping policemen and torture yourself and get through it and prevail and fill up that page! You must actually *love* the process, the struggle that complements your passion. The late great Pulitzer Prize-winning sports columnist Red Smith expressed this so eloquently when he said, "Writing a column is easy. You just sit at your typewriter until little drops of blood appear on your forehead." And without this toil, the rewards are not nearly so great, whether it's writing or whatever you do passionately.

It cracks me up when on occasion people tell me that my writing seems effortless. *If they only knew!* And now, if only I can find the inner strength to endure my present struggle and embrace it and survive it and find my way to . . . *the stars!*

I am seeing in my mind's eye the twelve inspirational words inscribed in the stone south pillar of Hopkins Memorial Gate at Williams College: "Climb High, Climb Far, Your Goal the Sky, Your Aim the Star." A lofty sentiment as far as the *astra* part goes, but what about the *aspera*? Guess they ran out of granite.

A few days later, I return to the same thought, that of finding inner strength in the midst of anguish. Looking out my window and daydreaming, my mind's ear is hearing the wonderful opening verse from a poem by Emily Dickinson:

A Wounded *Deer—leaps highest—*

I am imagining a wounded deer leaping high, over a fence perhaps or just into the sky, in an effort to escape to safety or as a reaction to its pain and heightened adrenaline. By extension, I know by experience (although now it is not so easy to put into practice) that we humans can also use our pain—physical and mental—to achieve more, or to be stronger or more motivated than we normally are. The power of motivation and the desire to overcome adversity both spring into action as a result of hardship and struggle. The next few days will be rough, for both me and Susan. Making it through the surgery, then awaiting The Verdict. And I will be a *Wounded* Deer, for sure, and will think often of Emily's five compelling words. Ah, the power of poetry.

Showtime. I finally meet Hyung Kim, my outstanding and skilled urologist and kidney surgeon. He tells me in his gentle yet strong voice that he has studied the biopsy results, and everything should be okay: he thinks the cancer cells haven't spread yet and that he can remove the tumor safely. Susan and I heave simultaneous gargantuan sighs of relief, knowing all too well, once again, that it's easier said than done. But if anyone can do it, it is Hyung.

Cut to the OR. All I am thinking about is that I must survive this and I must be strong, for Susan and my kids and my family members and my close friends and all the writing I have left to do and the twenty more years of life I have solemnly promised to Susan. First things first. This surgery, then the transplant, then getting better, then returning to my life again.

Before I go under, I am thinking about the tongue-in-cheek but wise counsel our old house painter in Brooklyn, Irv Sukenik, used to give me when I was in elementary school: "If you get out of this world alive, kiddo, you're lucky!"

Now I am contemplating this concept of luck: If I get out of the surgery, will I be lucky? That they found the tumor in its early stages? That they found it while they were testing me for a totally different reason? That I am here at all, considering that I am basically too old to be eligible for a heart transplant? Will it be luck, or simply being in the right place at the right time? Or do I just deserve to make it through this ordeal? Or is this just the way it's supposed to happen? Or . . . *hey, what do I know?*

Just before Hyung approaches me for his briefing and pep talk, I am hearing in my head one of my favorite songs ever, John Fogerty's "Centerfield." I love it so much, in fact, that I have chosen it as the ring tone on my iPhone. The chorus says so much about what I am feeling now, about getting back in the game, about potential and passion and desire:

> *Oh, put me in coach, I'm ready to play today*
> *Put me in coach, I'm ready to play today*
> *Look at me, I can be centerfield*

Hyung Kim is my coach now, in control of my fate. I need him to help me get back in the game. I'm ready to play. And I love the line *I can be centerfield.* I want to be back in the middle of all the action. *I can do it, coach!* (I also love the choice of the verb *be* in the final verse, as opposed to *play*, because—aside from rhyming with the preceding *me*—it implies total immersion and absolute identification with the position.) This feeling is so universal, as Fogerty sings so simply and poignantly at the end of the opening stanza (*Anyone can understand the way I feel*). And what's more, centerfield strikes a special, personal chord in me because the song mentions by name perhaps the three greatest centerfielders ever: Willie Mays, Ty Cobb, and Joe DiMaggio, all of whose talents I have long admired. Especially those of Willie, who was and will always be my favorite baseball player. He was, to me, the greatest all-around player of all time: best ever in all five "Leo Durocher" categories (hit, hit with power, run, field, throw); twenty-four All-Star games with 1.000 fielding percentage; intangible qualities of excitement, instinct, and flair; end of discussion. (I could go on and on, but I am going under and out very soon.)

Waiting for the anesthesiologist to approach, I am thinking of Susan, as I do every minute of every day. But especially now, as the phrase from our wedding vows echoes in my brain: "Till death do us part." *Nope,* I think. *Death will not us part. Not now.*

The final image that floats into my brain before I go under is the Sunday *New York Times* obituary column, which I've skimmed through for over fifty years. After reading a blurb and looking at the photo of the deceased, I invariably say to myself, "How sad" and "Lucky me." And now, here I am in the OR, awaiting my own fate. Will I soon be a blurb and a photo in the *Times*? Will people be reading about my demise over their coffee some Sunday morning in the very near future?

Will *they* be the ones looking at *my* picture—perhaps with that odd mixture of empathy and Schadenfreude—and saying, "How sad" and "Lucky me"?

8

What Do I Know?

Like a deus ex machina in some Greek tragedy, from somewhere above, the word comes down to save my sorry ass. After a day and a half of waiting anxiously following the surgery, Susan and I learn that, just as he had predicted and hoped, Hyung has successfully removed all the cancer from my right kidney, and . . . it hasn't spread! Phew to the nth. In short order, I am back on the 1A transplant waiting list, this time for a brand new heart *and* kidney.

The anticipation of it all! Remember the Carly Simon song "Anticipation"? Well, it has been playing in my head constantly throughout these past few days while I awaited The Verdict. As background music to the visual of the ketchup pouring oh-so-slowly in that old Heinz commercial.

Waiting around for crucial results is not my forte. And, I suppose, not for lots of people, either. Whether you are waiting for your grades on a report card or to hear from a college or university about acceptance or rejection or from your boss about getting a raise or a pink slip or for the results of an election or a Supreme Court decision or even to hear if you have won an Academy Award, it's never easy. But when you are waiting to get the decision regarding whether you will live or die, well, that's a horse (and hopefully not a hearse) of a different color.

While you're waiting to hear your fate, you could be thinking of your loved ones, and if you will either be leaving them behind forever or live to enjoy them for years to come. Or you could be thinking of all you have accomplished in your life and all you have failed to accomplish and all you have yet to accomplish. Or you could be thinking of how you can spend your waiting time preparing emotionally for the decision. Or you could be thinking of the challenging choice you have, when placed in such a dire situation, between trying to maintain control and letting go. Or you could be thinking of the provocative issues of luck and randomness. Or of the quandary of justice vs. injustice. Or of how life, like sports, is a game of inches and how little the margin is that separates a hit from a miss, a hero from a goat, success from failure, winning from losing . . . life from death. The implications of these concepts are so sad and could end up in tragedy. Or so compelling and could end up in triumph. In fact, I am thinking about all of these issues and possibilities. *A lot.*

And I am concluding that things will happen as they will happen (and maybe as they're supposed to happen, but the jury in my mind is still out on that thorny one). That—easier said than done—I can't worry about anything over which I have no control. That I must try with all my might to avoid cynicism. (The German aphorism expresses this feeling best: "*Das Leben ist wie eine Hühnerleiter—kurz und beschissen,"* "Life is like a chicken ladder—short and shitty.") That, finally, all I can do is to hope for the best and expect the worst. Or, as Doris Day so glibly sang it, "Que sera, sera."

Control and letting go. What a challenge. What a dilemma. Like most people, I assume, I like to be in control (of my schedule, of my plans, of my thoughts, of my life), but sometimes there's no way. I am musing about one of my favorite pet peeves and nemeses, SpellCheck, over which I have no control and which sometimes seems, alas, to have a mind of its own.

To wit: a college classmate of mine, Jim Kramer, and I now have new nicknames for each other, thanks to SpellCheck. I e-mailed him a while ago, and you must know how hard it is (on iPhones and computers) to get foreign—and other infrequently used—words past the eagle eye of SpellCheck. I was trying to share a memory with Jim about "wallball," a feverishly competitive game we used to play on the Chi Psi fraternity (later, the Spencer House) front porch at Williams. So when I typed *wallball*, SpellCheck (to whom "wallball" was obviously a stranger) substituted . . . *wallaby*! And then it did it a second time, then a third. At that point, I threw my proverbial hands up, and *wallaby* it remained. And then—salt in the wound—when I asked Jim to give a *bisou* (French for "kiss") to his wife, Judy (who was a French major at Bryn Mawr), freaking SpellCheck substituted . . . *bison*! I tried three more times, gave up, and *bison* it was. To my unmitigated dismay, I had lost complete control, but I really didn't care at that point. So from then on, I call Jim "Wallaby," and he calls me "Bison." Go figure: sometimes letting go can put a smile on your face.

Today, I am moved to a new, somewhat less depressing room down the hall on the fifth floor. Ironically, way out there but a million miles from my room, it features a gorgeous view of the Hollywood Hills, crowned by the iconic (and, now, ironic) HOLLYWOOD sign, symbol of glitz, glamour, high energy, and youth.

After the wonderful and uplifting news (Susan and I cried *plenty* when we heard) of the nephrectomy results, another sleeping policeman pops up on my road to survival: the tough recovery from the surgery, the pain and the angst, and, now that I am miraculously back on the transplant waiting list . . . the waiting!

Carbon-copy days go by, and paper-thin is my patience. Against my better judgment (actually, I've lost all sense of judgment by now), I have become testy and short with some of the nurses. I know deep inside that it is the pain and the impatience and the frustration that are the culprits (and my scapegoats), having taken their toll on my nice, friendly, civil side and replaced it, much of the time, with an unaccustomed and inappropriate Mr. Hyde.

After a few unpleasant encounters with RNs, I receive a visit from Michele Hamilton, Director of the Heart Failure Program and one of my staunch allies on the Committee to Decide My Fate. Michele is a very bright, very compassionate person, yet one who doesn't suffer fools gladly and is equipped with a hypersensitive bullshit detector. She gets right to the point.

"Listen, Bob, I hear that you've had a few, shall we say, 'encounters' with some of the nurses."

"Yeah, I guess I was a little curt with them, but sometimes they really piss me off—"

Daggers is too tame a word to describe the look she shoots me.

"I know, I know, they can sometimes be a pain, and I also think I know what you're going through. But listen to me. You'd better shape up and knock it off. Word gets back to the committee, and your chances of getting a new heart might well be jeopardized. It's not a big deal just to try and tone it down. But it *will be* a big deal if you don't."

I get the message, loud and clear, and promise to be more tolerant and sweet. The old "playing the game of politics and diplomacy while holding your figurative nose" gambit. Easier said than done, but I guess dodging another bullet isn't too much to ask of myself, considering what's at stake.

The next day, I receive a delightful visit from Susan and my older daughter (and middle child), Jenny, who has flown to the LA area on business from her home in Atlanta and who has dropped by to see her dear ol' dad.

Jenny has many great qualities, and among them are her maturity and judgment. It is particularly satisfying to me that both Susan and Jenny are advising me, in unison, to get with the program and be more cooperative with the nurses. Not only do I need to hear that, but I am thrilled that Jenny understands the situation so well, has the maturity and self-confidence to teach me—*her own father!*—a thing or two and to give me sage advice, daughter to Dad. I feel proud, not humbled. And I am feeling so good inside that not only Jenny, but Noah and Sarah, too, have turned out to be such good kids and such good human beings.

After the high of Jenny and Susan's visit, though, I am feeling terribly lonely once again and surrender myself, as usual, to
my thought processes.

Actually, it may sound funny, but thinking—along with love
and music—saved my life here at Cedars-Sinai. I don't know
what other patients do while waiting for a new heart to pop
up magically. For myself, unable to move around and without
the energy to write on my laptop and too tired to watch TV, I
naturally descend deep in thought, to escape Fear and Trembling and general insanity and to try to put this whole messy
and troubling and overwhelming experience into some sort of
perspective and to clarify things in my mind and to get my head
around what's happening to my heart and to bury myself in a
realm in which I feel comfortable and that I have cultivated my
entire adult life.

Plus, it feels way good.

As the existentialist French writer Jean-Paul Sartre once
opined, "If you are lonely when you're alone, you are in bad
company."

And here's the absolutely amazing and paradoxical and
ironic and meaningful thing about all this thinking that I did
throughout my one hundred days of being in the various hospitals: all the fruits of my thinking, all the lessons I learned, all the
learning I experienced about the human condition and about
life were forced upon me by my very imprisonment, by my horrendous ordeal, by the tests and trials and tribulations that my
dire and life-threatening condition foisted upon me, that the
circumstances of my life teetering on the brink and on the edge
of mortality compelled me to consider and to confront. In the

midst of complaining silently about or obsessing over physical pain or mental anguish or when this ordeal will ever ever end, I forced myself to think. Past the grim present, and into the past and the future and the abstract. About all the issues and conflicts that I had encountered during my checkered life. And oddly enough, this deep thought gave my horrific experience in the here-and-now great perspective, great clarity, and even great meaning, tempering my flaws with insights, my limitations with potential.

I have done this often, when the chips were way down, and it has, without fail, always seemed to be immeasurably helpful.

Speaking of which, one day during my recovery from the nephrectomy, an apt memory surfaces, of George Pistorius's seventeenth-century French class at Williams and philosopher Blaise Pascal's "thinking reed" quote: "Man is only a reed, the weakest in nature, but he is a thinking reed." Or, as his rival, René Descartes, said, "I think, therefore I am." I am obviously a sentient being, and feeling is something that I practice daily, hourly, every minute, every second. But now, in the midst of my pain and my waiting, thinking is coming in mighty handy.

And so, not surprisingly, I am deep in thought one Sunday morning, staring out my old friend, the window. I am struck by how fortunate I am to have escaped Death, at least so far, yet how luck doesn't really exist, *so what am I talking about?* And also by how, conversely, I deserve to have escaped Death and how it could've turned out the other way with me a goner and how unfair that would've been, yet how justice doesn't really exist, *so what am I talking about?* So here I am, lying in my bed on IV drips that are keeping my sick heart alive and depending on my brain to make sense out of all of this, and my brain is confused and conflicted and rudderless and clueless. *What do I know?*

I resume my internal monologue about luck and (in)justice, just to find some answers and to get back on my mental horse.

As usual, I begin with sports, the great metaphor for life. And like life, a game of inches. How many times the boundary between fair and unfair, and success and failure, is so tiny. A wisp of wind, a moment of hesitation, the slightest discrepancy of accuracy or timing, and either all is lost or to the victor the spoils! Take Billy Buckner's famous goof, for example. Ninety-nine percent of the time (at the very least), he surely would've caught Mookie Wilson's pathetic bleeder instead of letting it ooze through his legs. And yet, it did, and instead of being remembered as a terrific all-around first baseman, he is only remembered as the Goat of the 1986 World Series. How unfair is *that*? The same is true for Bobby Richardson's being at the right place at the right time to catch Willie McCovey's liner to end the 1962 World Series or Red Sox catcher Carlton Fisk's homer just staying fair (or unfair, if you rooted for the Reds) in the 1975 Series or a soccer or hockey shot just hitting the goalpost and missing being a goal by a centimeter and bouncing back into play or a potentially game-winning field goal in football doinking tragically off the crossbar or a tennis shot just nicking (or missing) the line or a golf ball plugging in a bunker or crawling into a divot or barely hitting the lower limb of a tree or a ball or a puck taking a crazy bounce or a ski or a skate or a sled hitting a hidden bump or imperfection. An inch or less one way or the other, and you're the hero and not the goat. Or vice versa, depending.

And then there's the whole issue of *Why me?*

This is such an easy trap to fall into, especially when we are very sick. Bad things do happen. And when they happen to us, paranoia might set in, and we might wonder why. Why me, instead of someone else? Was it somehow *meant* to be?

I am thinking of the story of Ralph Branca, the Brooklyn Dodgers pitcher who gave up that fateful (and, to me, wonderful) home run to Bobby Thomson in the 1951 third and deciding pennant game against my Giants. After the game, he is disconsolate and crushed, believing (wrongly, of course) that he alone was responsible for the Dodgers' mortifying loss.

As he is leaving the Polo Grounds, he meets his priest, Father Pat Rowley, with whom he discusses the "tragic" event.

"But why me, Father?" Ralph asks. "I love this game so much. Why did it have to be me?"

To which Father Rowley replies, "God chose you because He knew you'd be strong enough to bear this cross."

Now, I'm not a religious person, but this little story resonates with me, especially now. To me, the lesson to be learned is that the answer to "Why me?" is that it just happened to be me, not for any particular reason, and that when misfortune or adversity or extreme challenge (take your pick) strikes, we are obligated to be strong and to fight with all our might and to get through it somehow. Branca did, and he overcame the stigma and humiliation of what he did and took responsibility and carried on and led a good and happy life.

Of course, in my case, this is so ironic, because the story of Ralph Branca's life is quite inspiring to me, and yet he was in a strange way my hero in 1951, not because he was the person he was, but because his "blunder" allowed my Giants to win the pennant that year in such a dramatic and emotional way.

In the end, I believe that it is not a question of the luck of the draw, because if we take emotion out of the equation, we're left with an inch here and an inch there. In other words, we're left with the simple fact that something (bad) happened to happen, and you do what you can do with passion and grit, and the chips will fall where they may. Which probably evens out, with the outcome sometimes good, sometimes bad. And so, isn't "Why *not* me?" just as valid a question as "Why me?"?

Justice, injustice . . .

I am singing silent words from Gilbert and Sullivan's operetta *The Mikado*:

> *See how the Fates their gifts allot,*
> *For A is happy, B is not.*
> *Yet B is worthy, I dare say,*
> *Of more prosperity than A.*

Now I ask you, is that fair?

I am hearing in my brain Marlon Brando (Terry Malloy) in the back of the cab in *On the Waterfront* telling Rod Steiger (his brother, Charley), "I coulda been a contendah."

Of course, I am constantly tempted to ask, "Why me?" because according to life's "Rules of Justice," I don't "deserve" to have a sick heart: I have always been extremely fit, I have always had a pretty good diet (as an adult), I have never had a weight problem, I haven't smoked cigarettes in over forty-five years. Yet my dad had heart disease, so were it not for genetics . . .

In my dad's generation, in fact, the concept of justice was laughable and scorned. For instance, here's how our conversation would go down after my older brother got something and I didn't:

Me: "It's not *fair!*"

Dad: "*Life* isn't fair!"

But, if you think about it, life's not especially unfair, either.

The concept of injustice is odd, because it means the absence of justice, which may not exist in the first place. Is life basically unjust? Do we inevitably suffer, as Hamlet soliloquizes, "the slings and arrows of outrageous fortune"? Sometimes it seems that way, since we are much more sensitive when justice, a man-made concept, fails us when we ourselves fail. But when we succeed? Doesn't justice work in our favor then? Maybe it does, but then, we are much less aware of and preoccupied with it. Why should life be fair? Or unfair, for that matter? Maybe it just *is*. Maybe things just *happen*, period.

So if there is no injustice, what about the concepts of fate and destiny? Or even God? How do we explain life's mysteries and "miracles," if not by myths and belief systems that we create for ourselves? Or even sometimes by believing in arbitrary and certainly problematic entities like luck and justice? These are all, to me, man-made concepts that are employed, of course, by humans, especially in times of trouble, to help explain what is happening and why it is happening. The need for a higher force, wiser than we are, to help us in times of need. A shoulder to lean on. An explanation of life's big question marks. This is all well and good, for people who choose to follow this path.

On the other hand, life could simply be random, and what happens to us is either "meant to be" or, perhaps more plausibly, just occurs. After all, aren't God, fate, destiny, and (in)justice absolutes? And doesn't that mean that if we believe in them, we give up the control of our lives to that of something else, some higher force that is always right and just and true? And doesn't that mean that, for justice to work for us Americans, we should depend on and believe in and put our faith in the highest court in the land, the Supreme Court, to make unbiased, apolitical, objective decisions that will affect all our lives? Yes, surely that is what we should do.

Harrumph.

The alternative is existential and, to me, just as viable an option: shit happens, it just does, and it's how we deal with it ourselves that matters. A quote by the American writer Jack London (whose novels *The Call of the Wild* and *White Fang* I gobbled up and adored in sixth grade) sums it up: "Life is not always a matter of holding good cards, but sometimes playing a poor hand well."

A few days later, still waiting for my two organs, still unsure of how long I can go on with my very sick heart on IV life support and in such dire straits, still weak and in serious pain from the kidney surgery and completely disoriented, I am visited by a few cardiologists, who assure me that, based on their numbers and figures and statistics and algorithms, they know that everything is going to work out. *Know?* I respect their competence and love their optimism, but . . . *know?* And I am suddenly struck by a paradox that I began to be aware of in college, over a half-century ago, and that has been on my mind ever since the uncertainty of this whole cardiac ordeal began: How can we mere mortals know so much yet know so little? How can we be so in touch with what is happening and so aware of the nuances of the human condition, yet without a clue regarding both?

How can my docs really *know* what my fate will be? Is this knowledge based on empirical evidence, thus guaranteeing 100 percent certainty? Is it cockeyed (or rhetorical) optimism? Or is it a glib remark, a condescending reassurance, a mere . . . *manner of speaking?*

On the other hand, I am recalling a quote bequeathed to me by my amazing high school Latin and Greek teacher, the great Gil Feldman: the Greek playwright Menander's "*Lupes iatros estin anthropos logos*," "For man, knowledge is the physician of grief." Knowing helps you in virtually every aspect of life: excelling in your field of expertise; being aware of your environment; speaking intelligently with your family, friends, acquaintances, and colleagues; and being a good citizen and a good parent. To say nothing of finishing the *New York Times* Sunday crossword puzzle.

At the risk of seeming presumptuous, let me offer a piece of advice to all patients, whether you are in a doctor's office or, especially, in a hospital being bombarded with all kinds of tests and probes and you have a general idea of what's happening, but as far as the details go, you really don't have a clue and . . . *you need to know!* My humble tip: *Never hesitate to ask questions.* I am never shy about asking questions (as opposed to accepting blindly what doctors or nurses are telling me, a phenomenon I have witnessed all too often with others). I have to know all the details and what they mean and all the ramifications and what if this happens and why and what if that happens and why and what the side effects of this or that are. Otherwise, I am caught in the muck of ignorance and the mire of partial understanding, and that's not good. And besides, *Knowledge is the physician of grief!*

And this goes, I think, for most everything in life. Intellectual curiosity allows you to be enlightened and satisfied and educated and more knowledgeable and better prepared. Not to mention the fact that it lowers your stress and raises your awareness and your confidence.

One man who apparently didn't possess this thirst for knowledge was Wes Westrum, the catcher for the NY Giants of the 1950s. When he was managing the woeful Mets in the mid-'60s and they eked out a long extra-inning game, he was later grilled about the game by reporters.

"So, Wes, what are your thoughts about the game?" one journalist asked.

Wes scratched his head, thought a moment, and replied, "Well, it was a real cliff dweller."

I *know* how good my docs are. I *know* I'll get a new heart and kidney at some point. I *know* I'll make it through all this. Yep, knowledge is good!

I am reflecting on another advantage of the thirst for knowledge, that of bonding with another human being by sharing a common passion.

The most powerful example of this phenomenon in my life occurred during the summer of 1965. I am a twenty-year-old college senior-to-be, and I am spending that summer as a tennis counselor at Raquette Lake Boys Camp in the Adirondack Mountains of upstate New York.

The very first member of the RLBC staff I meet that summer is the baseball counselor, Kenny Horn. We bond instantly, partly because we share a passion for sports, especially baseball. We both happen to have a huge mass of mostly useless baseball trivia crowded into our temporal neocortices, and one of the ways in which we share this knowledge with each other is a game we call "Initials of the Fifties." Since we are both hyper-competitive (in a friendly way), this game is fierce, intense, and combative, as if our lives were at stake. And it goes something (actually, precisely) like this.

Kenny and I take turns uttering to his competitor two initials followed by a position and a major league baseball team of the 1950s in hopes that the recipient of the information will be unable to solve the riddle of who the player is. The pace is rapid-fire and the pressure nearly unbearable.

"B. P., pitcher, Redlegs," Kenny offers.

"Bud Podbielan," I answer immediately and proudly, then fire off my challenge.

"T. A., catcher, Pirates."

"Toby Atwell," Kenny ripostes punctually, a huge grin puffing up his cheeks.

"R. S., first base, Browns," he posits.

"Roy Sievers," I respond briskly.

And then: "C. P., outfield, Senators."

"Carlos Paula," Kenny answers in a trice, nailing it.

You get my drift.

Well, one hot afternoon after lunch, I run past Kenny on my way from the mess hall to the tennis courts and whisper in his ear, "R. R., pitcher, Cubs," then disappear up the hill. I see neither hide nor hair of him all day and into the evening.

At roughly 2 a.m., Kenny tiptoes into my tent (inhabited by me and the six campers for whom I am responsible) and whispers stealthily in my ear, "Robert Rush," awakening me from a deep sleep. "You bastard," he continues, as he has finally figured out that I had tried to bamboozle him by using *Bob* Rush's never-used formal Christian name, which was really against the unwritten rules of the game. And he exits my tent, leaving me startled, shamed, pissed off, and giddily happy, all at the same time. This was all part of our friendly competition, and the gleeful sharing of our common knowledge was the source of the bonding of our friendship, which remains, over fifty years later, strong to this day. Ah, the joys of knowledge!

And yet.

On the other hand (of "knowing"), there's the viewpoint of the sixteenth-century French essayist, Michel de Montaigne, who famously queried, "*Que sçais-je?*" or "What do I know?" Had it written in stone in his house and on a medallion hung around his neck. And this was an unspeakably brilliant and knowledgeable guy!

In my hospital bed, I am reflecting now on Montaigne, on reading and teaching him four decades ago, on the effect his writings have had on my life, on his attitude toward humility, which is the complementary side of knowing, the innocent honesty of admitting your ignorance and of being open to other points of view, and of learning. This is, incidentally, the same enlightened strategy employed by Confucius and Socrates. (On the contrary, this worthy philosophy isn't exactly what former NBA great Charles Barkley had in mind when he titled his memoir *I May Be Wrong but I Doubt It.*)

As it happens, the flip side of humility, going way back to Greek times, is hubris, which can't exist—ullage-wise, that is—without its opposite, humility, and vice versa. Hubris is the quality of feeling superior, of being arrogant (literally, of defying the gods). I am thinking now of two exemplars of hubris, King Oedipus and Victor Frankenstein. Eventually, people like them are punished for their hubris (the Greek concept of nemesis), it catches up with them, they are brought down to Earth, revenge and retribution are exacted, their nose is rubbed in it, they are hoist with their own petard.

Take me, for example.

I am recalling oh-so-vividly the advertising class I taught for nine years (with art director Seymon Ostilly, of "profound caca" fame) at the School of Visual Arts in New York City. The course, which meets one evening a week for three hours, is titled "Thinking 101," because great print ads are produced not by great writing or great artwork or great layouts or great typeface, but by great thinking. The students are all trying to put together portfolios to present to creative directors at ad agencies, who will hopefully be impressed by their work and hire them. The course has always been popular and has always drawn crowds.

It is November 1988, and I am giving the students a mini-lecture about the creative process. At one point, I am speaking about writing headlines and proffering my two Golden Rules (like the Oracle's), which I have attempted to drum into their heads unceasingly ever since the very first class a few months ago.

"Now don't forget, you guys: first, never, *ever* write a two-word headline; and second, don't *ever* try to be cute. No puns, no word plays, no pithy, coy, obtuse, quick sound bites. I promise you, from experience, these two rules will be invaluable to you as you sally forth in your advertising careers, and you can thank me later!"

A student way in the back row raises her meek little hand.

"We all know you've talked about this before, Bob, that thing about the two words, but can you explain once again why not?"

I bite my lip and formulate the words in my head carefully before responding to her. *Do my Official Pronouncements mean nothing to you? Are you not heeding my Wisdom from On High? Is it, for some inscrutable reason, not sinking in?*

Deep breath.

"Well, let me be clear," I respond with the patience of Job. "To write a good headline with a strong concept, you need a little room to express an idea intelligently. You need words that are clear, direct, intelligible, insightful, and also provocative. Words that are married to your visual in a symbiotic way, so that one can't exist without the other. To achieve all this, two words— with a few *extremely rare* exceptions, like Doyle Dane Bernbach's print ad for VW, Think Small—just aren't enough!"

Calm down, I am scolding myself. *She'll get it, maybe after the 1,548th time.*

The moment is finally here. *Judgment Day.* It's the part of the class when all the students—with great anticipation and high hopes—present their ads from the assignment of the previous week. The assignment for this week is simple yet deceptively difficult: execute (write and design) an ad about Bayer aspirin. Now, aspirin happens to be a preemptive category, or one in which there are no real differences between the brands (aspirin is aspirin), so the ad has to, in some way or another, stand out from the crowd by being provocative and memorable and fresh.

The students approach the two large side walls in the class-room and attach their aspirin ads with push pins, then take their seats. The walls are now filled to the brim with all kinds of ads that contain all manner of thinking. Seymon and I smile at each other proudly.

One by one and in order of their ads' positions on the wall, the students recount how they came up with their concepts and executions, hold up their ads, explain their visuals, read their headlines, and then await our criticism and, if they're very lucky, our praise.

The first six students present their ads, which range from abysmal to not terrible. Seymon comments on layouts, positioning, alternative visuals, media usage. I criticize word choice, tone, nuance, lack of simplicity or clarity, verbosity, coyness, and whether the headline is redundant or complementary in regard to the visual.

And then, without fanfare, student #7 steps up to the plate. She is a copywriter wannabe, and the ads she has previously presented in prior weeks have shown promise but have not particularly been jaw-droppers.

She proceeds to explain her ad with surprisingly sublime simplicity and directness: "This is an ad for Bayer aspirin," she begins. "I had just seen the musical *Les Misérables*, and I kept thinking about the title. So I came up with this ad. The visual is the musical's emblem, an etching of the waif Cosette, from Victor Hugo's novel. I changed the image so that her left arm is raised slightly, and I stripped into her hand a bottle of Bayer aspirin. The headline is . . ."

Seymon, the class, and I wait with hopeful anticipation.

"... Less Miserable."

Talk about jaw-droppers. Mine is on the floor.

Oh, the humility of it all! The ignominy! The shame! I had been drumming into these students' heads my irrefutable, written-in-stone Two Commandments of Headline Writing, again and again, with the certainty of knowing and the gravitas of a true believer, and what did this rank amateur and clueless tyro present to the entire class, and in my very presence? Why, nothing less than an ad with a headline that . . . contains two words and is also an outrageous pun!

And to make matters worse, the ad she presented, in my opinion, is absolutely brilliant! It seems so effortless, and yet I'm certain that she worked her ass off to come up with the concept. Talk about *sprezzatura!*

And to make matters even worse than that (is this *possible?*), she is the very same student who asked me to repeat my two Golden Rules of Headline Writing less than an hour earlier. Was she torturing me, like a malevolent character in a Poe short story, knowing full well that she had created an award-winning ad that broke into smithereens my Sacred Headline Rules?

So there I am, sitting on the desk at the front of the class, my jaw still on the floor, brought down to Earth by nemesis, revenge and retribution exacted upon me, my nose rubbed in it, the poster boy for the expression "hoist with his own petard." Yep, me: cocksure, arrogant, hubris-engorged Oedipus Mitchell!

After swallowing my considerable pride, I apologize sheepishly to the class and promise them (and myself) never again to be dogmatic and never again to prod and cajole them (and myself) to follow rigid rules. The great irony is that I am an inveterate believer that, when appropriate, the breaking of rules is one's absolute responsibility and even personal duty.

What do I know?

In my hospital bed, I am thinking, still, of Montaigne and of that humbling classroom memory. And how humbled I have been in this hospital, stripped to my very nakedness and vulnerability and core, my flaws revealed like open wounds. At the very end of his huge collection of essays, Montaigne says of us all: "And on the highest throne in the world, we still are sitting only on our own bottom."

Sitting on our own ass, indeed!

The very next day, I am sitting on my literal and figurative ass in my prison cell and again pondering the issue of humility, a lesson learned from Montaigne's "What do I know?"

A vivid memory naturally surfaces: my preparation during my senior year at Williams for the upcoming Woodrow Wilson Fellowship interview. Doesn't mean much to me now, but back then, it was a big freaking deal. Getting this prestigious grant— which paid your way through graduate school—required filling out a lengthy application including your undergraduate scholastic record and recommendations from professors at your college or university, having it reviewed thoroughly by a Foundation board, and then, if you were fortunate enough to be chosen as a finalist, undergoing a sadistically tough interview at one of the regional academic campuses. It was essentially, at this point, the interview that could make or break you.

My preparation for the interview was divided into two parts, the biggest of which was boning up on my chosen subject for graduate study—French language and literature. For weeks, I spoke French to myself in private—in the shower, walking to class, wherever. And I read everything I could get my hands on that I hadn't read yet as an undergrad: poetry, prose poetry, novels, theater, philosophy, religious thought, scientific tracts, the whole *shmeer*.

The second part was attending individual biweekly meetings with a special Woodrow Wilson faculty adviser (a member of the Williams faculty). These meetings were extremely helpful and rigorous, consisting of his quizzing me about my specialty, discussing the comportment and obligations to which a Wilson scholar had to adhere, and (most important) being aware of the kinds of questions to expect from the interviewers.

At one point during a meeting with my adviser, he is giving me a piece of advice about answering questions during the interview.

"*I know* are two useful words that will serve you well throughout your life," he tells me. "But, funny enough, *I don't know* are sometimes equally useful."

When I return to my room, I am digesting this piece of advice. First, of course, I think of the Descartes/Montaigne dichotomy of knowing vs. not knowing. But for me, the concept of questioning one's (my) knowledge, at that time in my life, is pretty tough meat to digest, and easy to choke on: the mature, thoughtful person in me considers it to be very wise counsel, while the supremely confident, ultracompetitive whippersnapper of a twenty-one-year-old undergrad asshole in me demurs.

I'm not gonna say "I don't know" during this interview, I convince myself. *That would mean admitting defeat. I am really ready for this, and if I don't know the exact answer to a question, I surely know enough to make some sense out of it.*

Fast-forward to Cambridge, MA. I have just arrived on the Harvard campus for my long-awaited interview. I am a bit bedraggled, because I had driven the day before from Williams in a classmate's tiny VW Beatle smushed together with him and three other undergrads who are also fellowship candidates in different fields of study, got caught in a snowdrift during a horrendous blizzard, arrived at Harvard that afternoon three hours late for the interview only to discover to my (further) distress that it had been postponed until the next day because of the inclement weather, stayed overnight at a cheap hotel in Cambridge, got an hour of sleep total, and appeared in the interview building dressed in the same crushed shirt, pants, tie, and jacket I was wearing the day before.

The interview finally occurs and is going rather well, as I recall. The panel of interviewers (three or four of them, I think) is cordial and extremely pleasant and asks me a barrage of questions that are pretty tough, but nothing I can't handle. Why do I deserve a Wilson? What is the role of higher education, broadly speaking? Who wrote the poem "Vénus Anadyomène"?

Ever more self-confident, I calmly await the next query. There are only a few minutes left in the interview now, so how tough can this one be? *Time to wrap things up,* I am thinking, *so throw me softball, just for fun.*

"So, Mr. Mitchell," one of my interlocutors begins, his voice whispery and stately and dripping with pseudo-British gravitas. "Tell me, what does the French expression *la petite mort* mean?"

Holy crap. You kidding me? Why, of all the dirty, rotten, low-down . . .

My self-confidence is melted instantly like the Wicked Witch of the West, not by a bucket of water, but by my own petard. A textbook case of hubris.

My mind must recover from the shock, and *stat*. I am on the verge of panic but trying like hell to maintain the little equilibrium I have left in me. Problem is, despite all the French crammed into my hippocampus, *la petite mort* isn't something I have ever stored there.

Let's see, I am saying to myself, *"la petite mort." Sounds so simple. Damn! Er, "la petite mort," or "little death." Some kind of near-fatal injury? A stillborn child?* I'm fluent in French, have lived there and conversed with lots of people, have read French literature pretty widely. So why haven't I ever heard this expression uttered by voice or pen?

The seconds fly by . . . fifteen . . . thirty. An exceedingly long and mortifying pause. The interviewer is looking straight at me, a compassionate smile pasted on his angelic face. I am stumped. *Hey, is this a trick question?*

Now is the moment of truth. Or of lie. Dare I avoid defeat by taking an educated guess at this seemingly simple query? Shall I take a stab and answer, supremely confidently of course, that "La Petite Mort" is one of Baudelaire's earlier yet little-known (especially to the panel of judges) poems? That "little death" refers to the description of the demise of Napoleon— who was short in stature—by some novelist, maybe Hugo or Balzac? Or—

Suddenly and without warning, an Angel of Mercy swoops in, deus ex machina-like, and saves me. Piercing through my armor of invincibility and youthful stubbornness and pride, the memory of my Wilson faculty adviser's wise counsel about honesty and integrity saves me in the nick of time.

"I . . . I don't know," I respond in meek resignation.

"That's okay," my gracious interlocutor says. "We can't be expected to know everything." He continues, "Actually, *la petite mort* is a colloquial French expression meaning 'orgasm,' suggesting the feeling of weakness or faintness after the act."

I grin stupidly, both out of appreciation of the clever quaintness of the phrase and from the humiliation at not having known the answer.

"I had a French girlfriend during my sophomore year," I blurt after some thought, "but—pardon the expression—the phrase never came up."

My interviewer smiles wickedly, as do the other panelists acknowledging the cleverness of my double-entendre.

After the interview is over, I am feeling chastened but relieved. To this day, I have never forgotten that seminal (so to speak) moment in my young life, and my college adviser's sage tip to say *I don't know* when, well, I don't know. Not only am I pretty sure that this humility played a small part in my being chosen for the Wilson, but, much more important, it has stood me in great stead in many situations throughout my life and has helped teach me the importance of honesty, humility, and integrity.

As it happens, months after the interview, I spy a B. C. cartoon in the paper that reminds me of this experience and that causes me to guffaw silently. It is a drawing of a worm looking up at and reading a sign stuck in the ground.

The sign says, No WRIGGLING.

All of this to say that sometimes *I don't know* can be the three most important words you can own in your vocabulary. Aside from *I love you* and, of course, *Dewey Defeats Truman.*

Knowing, not knowing. Still lying in pain and limbo, I am ruminating—out of nowhere (well, perhaps my subconscious)—with more hope than ever before, on my new heart. At last, I am convinced that I *know* (from my gut), as my cardiologists do (from their heads), that my story will have a happy ending. Will I endure?

I know I can. I know I can.

And I sing to myself the melancholy yet prayerful words of the Tin Man from *The Wizard of Oz* (my present alter ego), which, I now realize, bizarrely and anachronistically suggest open-heart transplant surgery:

> *I could stay young and chipper*
> *And I'd lock it with a zipper*
> *If I only had a heart.*

9

That Good Night

Yesterday, a twenty-nine-year-old male was the victim of a fatal car accident. But oddly and miraculously, this very horrible tragedy has a very happy ending.

A helicopter whirs high above my hospital window. The RN chirps to me, "Hey! That's your new heart and kidney about to land!" After more than three excruciating months of waiting with varying degrees of patience, Susan and I gaze up at the chopper, then into each other's eyes. We are not sure whether to laugh or cry or what. I'm not usually an overtly emotional person, but my eyes are glistening, a shiver rattles my spine, the hair behind my neck stands at attention, and a lump forms in my throat, a lump bigger than the malignant tumor they removed from my kidney. A single chubby tear rolls down Susan's cheek.

Ohmygodohmygodohmygod.

July 27, 2015, is now, officially, my second birthday.

The unfortunate victim happened to be at the wrong place at the wrong time. And I, at the right place at the right time.

A game of inches.

Within minutes, I receive congratulatory visits from several members of my amazing team of cardiologists: Dael Geft, Michelle Kittleson, Michele Hamilton, David Chang, Jon Kobashigawa, and Jig Patel. Then one from Irene Kim, the wonderful young surgeon who will soon be attaching a total stranger's kidney inside my abdomen.

And, last but not least, from Alfredo Trento, eminent thoracic and cardiac surgeon, The Man Himself, the person who, in a few hours, will be holding my sick heart in his talented hands and replacing it with a new one. He enters my room, and we chat in Italian for four minutes and thirty-three seconds, which must be a world record for him. (He is a superbusy guy: I am told that his patient visits usually last about eighteen seconds.) I am certain that the length and vitality of our discussion are due to the fact that he is Italian (from Padua) and I am fluent in his native language, which phenomenon, in my experience, is always a guaranteed recipe for immediate bonding.

At the end of our chat, I say to Alfredo, "*In culo alla balena,*" the Italian equivalent of "Break a leg." (Literally and charmingly, it means, "In the whale's ass": don't even ask.) Acknowledging my use of an insider's colloquial expression, he smiles kindly and winks, and I know in my gut that he has my back. And, more important, my front.

After he leaves, I am ruminating on how fortunate I am to be fluent in French and Italian. Throughout my adult life, this ability has enabled me to appreciate fully the culture, literature, popular music, and true essence of both countries and has facilitated my meeting and becoming close friends with a number of extraordinary people who are "natives." And now, it has allowed me to establish a rapport with the man who will, quite literally, be holding my fate in his hands.

As I await the nurses who will escort me to the OR, my mind, inspired by the chat with Alfredo, transports itself to Italy.

Ah, l'Italia!

I love everything about this country. And so does Susan. We have been returning there most every September for years. We just can't get enough of the regions and the cities and the villages and the vistas and the hills and the hidden vineyards and the monuments and the churches and the music and the art and the food and the wine and the coffee and the language and the customs. And especially the people.

There is something about the Italians that we love so much, especially the ones we have been fortunate enough to meet and befriend. And their friends and families. Now, we have met great people from a number of other countries, but the Italians—maybe it's their joyousness or their creativity or their sweetness or their optimism or their pizzazz or their love of life—there's just something quite special about them.

I am reflecting on all the great times we have spent in Italy with our dear friends Giuseppe and Maria (who live in Rome), Tania and Marco (Le Marche), and Mauro and Antonella (Venice). All the laughing and the shmoozing and the drinking and the eating and the walking and the photo taking and the hugging and the kissing and especially the friendship.

Damn, I wish we were there now . . .

But now, instead of an Alitalia Boeing 777 picking me up, here comes my old pal, the humble gurney, manned by the nurses who will trundle me off to meet my fate (and hopefully not my maker).

I am weak, exhausted, beaten up thoroughly by the IV drips that have been coursing through my veins for many months now, and, frankly, deep inside, *scared shitless*. But oddly, trumping all of these feelings are the hope and excitement of being on the threshold of a brand new life.

I purse my lips, grit my teeth, and slither my way with difficulty onto the narrow transport. I am cushioned by two extra pillows and warmed by two blankets and the loving companionship of Susan.

I am wheeled down the hallways of the sixth floor, negotiating the eight dreaded sleeping policemen I know by heart from all the lugubrious trips to the cath lab (for biopsies and Swan-Ganz procedures) and the x-ray and ultrasound rooms. When we reach the automatic doors leading to the OR, Susan and I say our brave and tender good-byes.

"See you in about twelve hours, sweetie," I say, brimming with optimism.

"You *will*, I *know* you will, my love," she says with conviction, looking deep into my eyes.

"I know it, too. As General MacArthur once said—"

"I *shall* return," Susan interrupts, intimately in touch with how my brain works.

We exchange loving glances, then I whisper, "It's gonna be okay, honey."

"I'm sure it will be," she says sweetly, adding an affectionate Italian expression that we whisper to each other every night just before we call it a day: "*Sogni d'oro!*"

Golden dreams, indeed.

Cut (sorry!) to the OR. Lying inert on the operating table, I look at the clock on the wall, and it reads noon on the dot.

The surgical team, milling about, is organized and purposeful, like a disciplined squadron of bees in a hive. As they prepare and attend to the surgical equipment, the anesthesia, the intubation devices, the lighting, and the monitors, each has a specific role and function. I appreciate what they do, obviously, because right now they are working like hell to save my life. And I admire and respect them, because they are doing what they do with engagement and efficiency and passion.

Passion is the key to true satisfaction and happiness, I am thinking. *If you do anything without passion, what good is it, huh?* This notion has always been, as long as I can remember, one of the guiding mantras of my life, a concept I have believed in steadfastly for myself and that I have tried to inculcate in my kids. (I guess they must have listened to me, since they all turned out to be pretty passionate people.)

I am recalling the twelve years of commuting to my work in advertising during the '80s and early-'90s, the daily hour-or-so train ride to New York City from Chappaqua, NY. And all the faces I used to observe in all the rows of the car I was in, faces buried in the *New York Times* or the *Wall Street Journal* or various forms of paperwork (this was way before laptops and iPhones), robotic faces that looked glum or bored or even comatose and that belonged to people who apparently had little passion for their work and, for that reason, must have been oppressed by it.

Now I am draped, shaven, disinfected, and otherwise thoroughly prepped for the twelve-hour ordeal to come (prep, heart transplant, intermission, prep, kidney transplant, cleanup). During the prepping process, I am left alone with my thoughts; and although the anesthesiologist will be approaching in just a few short minutes, I am forcing my mind to escape and drift away serenely to other places and times. And, of course, since the mind is a powerful thing, mine manages to stuff into this small pocket of time a massive torrent of thoughts, feelings, words, memories, and images.

I close my eyes and envision the clinically gruesome Rembrandt painting *The Anatomy Lesson of Dr. Nicolaes Tulp*, which I had first seen in a slide as a Williams freshman in my Art 101 class and then in person, many decades later, in the Mauritshuis museum in The Hague. A certain Dr. Tulp, the city anatomist of Amsterdam, is giving an anatomy lesson on the canvas. The corpse belongs to Aris Kindt, who was hanged earlier that day for the crime of armed robbery. The images in the painting are cascading back to me from long ago: the chiaroscuro, with light bathing the patient's body, especially the chest area (even though it is the corpse's left arm that has been cut open, the muscles and tendons exposed); Kindt's navel in the shape of a capital *R*, which stands for Rembrandt (or, in my case, Robert); the seven medical professionals surrounding the body. (Coincidence or not?: there are seven members of the surgical team now surrounding *me!*)

Opening my eyes, I am trying really hard not to focus on the physical reality of what is about to occur here shortly: my breastbone will be severed, my rib cage opened up, my useless and moribund heart removed from my body, and the spanking-ish-new heart attached via the left atrium, aorta, pulmonary artery, and both venae cavae. *Oy.* I have been under the knife before many times, but . . . *this is different.*

With no warning, I am filled with an overwhelming spurt of optimism, spawned not only by my fierce determination to live, but also by my total confidence in the cardiology team that has surrounded me for three months and, now, in Alfredo and his team in particular. Losing control of my life is not particularly my forte, but if I am forced to surrender my fate to someone else, this alone is the very time and place. A wise passage from Lao-tzu's *Tao Te Ching* springs to my mind:

> *Do your work, then step back.*
> *The only path to serenity.*

I am as calm as I could possibly be under the circumstances.

Yet, in addition to my determination and unexpected tranquillity, I am also feeling mighty humbled. Here I am, naked and vulnerable, my life on the line, a seventy-year-old guy with a bum ticker, a speck on the planet feeling the smallness of being a mere mortal. Now, closing my eyes once more, I am contemplating the times through the years when I felt this same human smallness in the universe as I stood in front of, inside, or under the grandeur of awesome art and architecture: the Amiens cathedral, Bosch's *The Garden of Earthly Delights* in the Prado, Michelangelo's statue of Moses in the San Pietro in Vincoli church and his ceiling in the Sistine Chapel, Rodin's statue *La Main de Dieu* in his eponymous museum, Gaudí's Basilica de la Sagrada Familia, Le Mont-Saint-Michel . . .

My thoughts wander to another humbling experience I often had that drove home to me my smallness in the cosmos: my encounter with the spectacular marine life of Maui. I spent many hours scuba diving in the 1990s on the back side of Molokini, a small horseshoe-shaped crater off the southwestern coast of the island. Being eighty feet beneath the surface of the water can sure do funny things to the ego: cruising among the manta rays, sea turtles, eels, fishes, corals, nudebranchs, anemones, and especially white-tip sharks gives a body the decided feeling of relative insignificance in the presence of such a glorious and awesome panoply of marine creatures.

And now, memories are wafting briskly into my mind in the form of a minidocumentary of my life, punctuated by sporadic cinematic fades and cuts. And in chronological order, as if in a résumé. My brain is summoning these particular recollections, probably because they represent a jumble of intense feelings that are woven tightly into the rich tapestry of my life. Feelings good and bad—like passion, hope, humility, and fear. The very same feelings I am experiencing now, simultaneously, lying helplessly here in the OR, frozen in time and space, and awaiting a new heart, a new life.

Fade up to a frigid winter night in Brooklyn, NY, 1955. Eleven-year-old me is lying in bed, listening to a basketball game between my beloved New York Knicks and the hated Syracuse Nationals. In a bold, curfew-defying act of derring-do to hide the sound and the deed from my parents, I have—stealthily, pre-meditatedly—tucked my tiny black plastic Emerson transistor radio (you know, the one with the lint-catching slits and the gold lettering and the teeny dials, just out on the market) underneath my pillow. I turn the volume up slightly in order to hear through the foam. Not too much, though—could get caught. There, just right. My ear is pressed hard against the pillow, and I am feigning innocent slumber, quiet as a small rodent, in case a parent should appear, unannounced, to check in on me. I am living, on the edge, the life of some escapee like Lt. Dunbar clinging to the top of the water tank from the inside in the film *Stalag 17*.

There I lie, little Bobby Mitchell, rooting my ass off for my pathetic NY Knicks, yelling silently like a lunatic, passionate, sweating bullets, my heart pumping like a Ft. Wayne piston, begging them for a victory. The Knicks are sucking, as usual, but they have mounted a fierce comeback and have forged ahead by two over the Syracuse Nats with three seconds to go in the game. I am lullabied by the sharp, rich, frenetic voice of the legendary announcer Marty Glickman: *Now it's Tricky Dick McGuire passing the ball to Braun on the right sideline. Carl feeds it to Harry "The Horse" Gallatin under the basket, then to Sweetwater Clifton. Now Sweets pushes it back to Braun at the top of the key for a two-handed pop shot . . . Gooooood . . . like Nedick's! And the Knicks finally take the lead, 82-80!*

Yay!

But then, as always, the Knicks blow it in the final seconds: *Now it's Dolph Schayes receiving a pass from Seymour, he slices sharply to his right, he drives past Gallatin, he lays it up, it's good, and he's fouled!*

Shit!

Schayes cans the winning foul shot, natch, and my hopes are, as usual, dashed. But I do love my passion and my loyalty and my innocent, infinite hope: there's always tomorrow, when they're gonna kick Rochester's ass!

Cut to the Williams College campus, October, 1962. I am a freshman and in the middle of a grueling soccer practice. A daily refuge from the intense academic grind, the soccer pitch at Cole Field is my second home, a little patch of paradise surrounded by the magnificent Berkshire foothills.

Oh, the Great Pyramid of Giza is fine, and the Hanging Gardens of Nebuchadnezzar will do. But in the full flush of autumn, the flaming countryside of Williamstown, MA, is the place to be for Wonder seekers. The foothills are miraculous conflagrations of leafy color, featuring patches of gold, then rust, then russet, then orange and scarlet and crimson and yellow brown and reddish brown and vermilion. Magic sprouted from majestic, effulgent stands of indigenous timber. Speckled Alder. Witch Hazel. American Beech and Yellow Birch. Basswood, Sumac, White Ash. Trembling Aspen. Largetooth Aspen. Late-changing Red Oak. Bird's-eye Maple and Moose Maple. Not to mention the ineffable lemon yellows of the coniferous Tamarack.

I am loving the pure joy of the workout in this cozy cocoon of beauty and intimacy—the spirited engagement, the feverish competition, the feeling of camaraderie and teamwork with my loyal and caring teammates (Upton, Caine, Urmy, Prozeller, Noll, Willett, Tobis, et al.). Even the pain of the warm-ups, the wind sprints, the running laps, the seriously excruciating calisthenics. God, was I fit then. *And, yes, invincible!*

And yet.

Fade to January, 1963, four months into my freshman year. I am sitting at my dorm room desk in front of my tiny green Olivetti Lettera 22 manual typewriter, casting a blank stare at the appropriately blank piece of typing paper that is peeking up defiantly above the rubber roller. And from out of the Berkshire blue, in creeps the pernicious shadow of self-doubt. *What ever happened to the confidence I'd been exuding since September? What the hell is Kant talking about? What is the meaning of Ingmar Bergman's* The

Magician, *that cockamamy movie I just saw on Spring Street? What language is Faulkner speaking? What language is my organic chemistry textbook speaking? Am I some impostor masquerading as a Williams undergrad? Fer chrissakes, who the hell am I?*

Cut to the seventies and eighties, now rushing through my brain, one scene of my three kids growing up fading softly to the next. Sarah and Jenny and I collecting gorgeous fallen leaves and gluing them artfully onto sheets of multicolored construction paper. The uproarious "King Pop" bedtime stories (starring King Pop, Queen Peep, Prince Poop, and Princess Pep) that I concocted for Noah, then for the girls. Spirited catches in the driveway with Sarah and Jenny and coaching them in basketball and softball. Watching Noah perform intensely at his karate dojo. Almost losing him to a sudden attack of acute epiglottitis in the wee hours. Teaching the kids vitally important linguistic factoids like which two words contain all the vowels in order (*abstemiously, facetiously*) and which word has three consecutive double letters (*bookkeeper*).

Cut to November, 1994. I am driving from Chappaqua to Berkeley, CA. (After spending most of the year in Tel Aviv teaching and lecturing on commercial TV writing and production and going through a divorce from my first wife, I make the decision to leave advertising, move to Berkeley, and start life anew, under the sun and not far from the ocean.) I am in my little red Mazda Miata after three grueling days of driving, having stopped for the first two nights in Joliet, IL, and Cheyenne, WY. It is 10 p.m., and I am driving scarily slowly, maybe 3 mph, in a ferocious blizzard on Interstate 80 at 7,000 feet through the Donner Pass. (Nope, happily, I wasn't then acquainted with the story of the cannibalistic Donner Party.) The visibility is about two feet, and I am nearly crashed into by a wobbling eighteen-wheeler. I am exhausted, physically and mentally, from the harrowing drive and frozen by the twenty-degree temperature and the fear. Somehow, I (barely) see an exit sign, semiblindly hobble my way to a Motel 6, check in, and flop onto my lumpy bed and two-inch-thick pillow.

Fade to the next morning, when I awake to realize that I am in the deserted town of Winnemucca, NV *(Winnemucca, Nevada?)*, that here I am, on the morning of my fiftieth birthday, in a Motel 6 in frigging Winnemucca, Nevada, having escaped multiple near-death experiences the night before and about to begin a new life in California, at the age of fifty, recently divorced and alone, with no idea of what I'm going to do in life, no friends within three thousand miles of the vicinity, no place to live, no belongings aside from a duffel bag brimming with clothes and books, my four tennis racquets, and my Martin guitar. I am nervous, humbled, and disoriented. Talk about a midlife crisis!

Cut to 1996 and John Newcombe's Tennis Ranch in New Braunfels, TX. I think I just died and went to heaven. I am spending six days of grueling, intensely competitive tennis there playing with and against sixty-three other accomplished players. And there to root us on—we are divided into four teams: the Musclemen, the Dunnies, the Wankers, and the Lawnmowers—are ten icons of the game of tennis (John Newcombe, Ken Rosewall, Roy Emerson, Tony Roche, Fred Stolle, Mal Anderson, Cliff Drysdale, Charlie Pasarell, Marty Riessen, and Owen Davidson), whose various roles are to hit with us, coach and ballboy for us, rib and ridicule us, encourage and instruct us, and stay up with us till the wee hours drinking Foster's and discussing the good ol' days.

In one of the deciding matches of the six-day team competition, I am up against a Brit solicitor, Howard Rogg (a great competitor and still a friend). Lots of fun, lots of pressure. The good news: even though he gets every goddam ball back, I am confident I can beat him. The bad news: I am handicapped, because on the second day here, I tore my right calf muscle, which—despite magical first aid applied valiantly and hourly by former Cincinnati Reds trainer Larry Starr (electric shock treatment, taping from ankle to knee, ice packs, and applications of Flexall 454 ointment, otherwise known as "Hot Stuff")—has rendered me gimpy and limpy, a Chester-from-*Gunsmoke* impressionist, and able to run at about 4 percent of my normal capacity.

So I drag my ass and bionic taped-and-iced-and-electrified right leg to the Rogg match, bowed but unbroken. After pulling my right hamstring in the third game (I am now taped up from ankle to *groin*), I limp around furiously and am forced to resort to frequent drop shots and topspin lobs and moonballs. I am beginning to figure Howard out. Miraculously, by using my tennis IQ and my shot repertoire (if not my crippled leg), I'm leading 5-3 and on my way to a heroic victory. But, alas, the disability and the pain get the better of me, reality sets in, and I proceed to lose ten of the next eleven games, dropping the match, 5-7, 1-6. But not without a dogged fight: many of the games go to thirty-all, some to eight or ten deuces. After the final point, I am utterly spent. The pain shooting through my right leg feels like an admixture of a coronary infarction, kidney stones lodged in my ureter, and (so I am told) childbirth. Ten minutes later, sitting in the gazebo, I am filled with joy and pain and pride and humility, all at the same time. I am not used to losing, but all that matters is that I gutted it out, for me and my teammates, and gave it everything I had, leaving it all there out on the court.

Cut to Santa Barbara, CA. It is June 10, 2001. I have moved here from Paris in April, and this morning I meet my soul mate, the love of my life, a woman (aptly) named Susan Ellen Love. She is an accomplished artist, working on the side as the head of the gift department at a local gourmet market, the one where Oprah shops for groceries. I enter the store in search of a grapefruit spoon. We meet and chat raptly for forty minutes. (I end up buying a grapefruit knife.) I call her up the next day, and we go out on our first date, a long walk on a gorgeous local beach. We chat so intensely and for so long that we lose track of the time and end up at a nudist colony. That evening, we return from dinner to my rented house and engage in a passionate first kiss. I experience an arrhythmia, my defibrillator shocks me, and I crash to the floor in a daze. Susan is also in shock, certain that her kiss has killed me and that she has, unwillingly and unwittingly, become a murderess.

Cut to Italy, September 2009. Susan and I are in Venice for four days, and she falls in love again (this time with Venice). As an artist, she is adoring—and madly taking pictures of—all the magic: the canals, the narrow streets, the bridges, the reflections on the water, the colorful laundry hanging outside, the doors, even the doorknobs. We spend four more days in Rome with our wonderful and dear friends, Giuseppe and Maria. Then four days in Umbria. The highlight is our stay at an inn, Il

Borgo dell'Ulivo, in the village of Matigge di Trevi, featuring an incredible twenty-two-course dinner (part of which is cooked over a humongous open bed of hot coals) planned by our host, master chef and friend of Giuseppe and Maria, Maurizio Bastianelli. We drink and laugh and chat and drink and have the best time together. At the end of the meal, we are all stuffed, sated, and *soddisfatti*, with food and friendship. Life is good.

Cut to Southern California, April-July, 2015. My mental camera now projects the final series of scenes, quick cuts shuttling from one medical event to the next: the five VT attacks, the EMTs rushing me to the ER, the life-support paraphernalia, the four hospitals, the bone marrow biopsy, the kidney cancer surgery, the gurney trip with Susan to the OR on my way to the transplant surgery—

Fade to black, my eyes open, and my mind returns from the documentary to reality. The Moment has finally arrived. I am realizing that, of all my seventy-plus years on Earth and all my memorable and significant experiences good and bad, this moment is, by about a million miles give or take, the most crucial and meaningful. Yep, this is *The Moment* I've been training for all my life.

The anesthesiologist approaches, I don my mask (or, rather, it is donned for me by a tech), and the soporific gas is introduced slowly into it.

Perchance to dream . . .

I am beginning to feel the grip of the potion and am pondering the frailty and the tenuousness of existence. I recite to

myself the familiar words from the Macbeth soliloquy about
life:

> *It is a tale*
> *Told by an idiot, full of sound and fury,*
> *Signifying nothing.*

As my nostrils sniff the gas as lovingly as Ferdinand the Bull's
sniff his flowers under his favorite cork tree in the 1938 Disney
film, I recite to myself the opening verses of the Dylan Thomas
villanelle:

> *Do not go gentle into that good night,*
> *Old age should burn and rave at close of day;*
> *Rage, rage against the dying of the light.*

The words were meant for his dying father, but, by telepathy,
I know that right now, they are also meant for me.

I am feeling my inner rage, and it is not one of hate, but of
defiance. I will *not* let Death conquer me. I will come out of
this better than ever. I repeat the phrase "that good night" and
consider how it intimates the peaceful darkness of death in the
poem. Funny, I am thinking, but the anesthesia is about to be
"that good night," too, a darkness that will render the potential
pain of the surgery peaceful. Yes. *My* good night is the anesthesia, and not Death. In the poem, Thomas refers to all kinds of
men—"wise," "good," "wild," "grave"—and how they did not
achieve all the things they wanted to, which compels them to
"Rage, rage against the dying of the light" and fight for their
lives. I am hearing you, Dylan, *and that is me now.*

In my gathering stupor, I am—for pure pleasure, and for auld lang syne perhaps—visualizing the most delicious steaks I've ever eaten and will never eat again (in addition to sushi and grapefruit, medium-rare meat is now forbidden to me forevermore, which is why this might have been one of my final—bittersweet—thoughts before going under): the sirloin at Joe Marsh's Spindletop in New York City (I was twelve), the porterhouse at Peter Luger in Brooklyn, the New York strip at Morton's in Palm Beach, the ribeye at Mandelbaum and Birnbaum in Tel Aviv, the *bistecca alla fiorentina* at Le Fonticine in Florence, the *pavé de salers* at La Reine Margot in Aurillac.

I am pretty much out of it now. But just before I am transported to la-la land (how strange, since I am already in LA) and drift away into the ether of nothingness, a final quote—this time from the great Latin orator and polymath Cicero—expels itself from my now-addled brain: *"Dum spiro spero,"* "As long as I breathe, I hope," which I have long loved not only for its meaning, but also for its euphony.

And now, as I segue gently from charcoal gray to black and teeter at the threshold of the abyss, I repeat the phrase, each time caressing every letter, the consonants in particular, and rejoicing in the passion of the sentiment:

Dum spiro spero . . . Dum spiro spero . . . Dum spiro spero . . .

10

The Heart Has Its Reasons

The light at the end of the tunnel is blinding: I made it!

I am lying on my beautiful, wonderful, newly made bed in the ICU. I am barely awake and definitely not with it. My foggy mind—not there, yet there—is drifting about, rudderless, on a sea of painkillers. I am aware of nothing but my random thoughts. My weary eyes are closed.

I thought I could.

Echoing in my mind, this phrase stirs a memory that has been lying fallow for close to seven decades.

I am really young, two maybe, and my mom is reading me Watty Piper's *The Little Engine That Could*, written in 1930, the classic story of the plucky little blue engine who, against all odds, pulled the long, stranded train with the goodies for the little boys and girls over the mountain by the sheer force of its determination. Mom is now reading me—with her trademark calm, lilting, and tender tones—the powerful and inspiring ending:

> *And the Little Blue Engine smiled and seemed to say as she puffed steadily down the mountain. "I thought I could. I thought*

I could. I thought I could. I thought I could.
I thought I could.
I thought I could.

I smile broadly when she finishes and ask—no, demand—
that she read it one more time. And now, some sixty-eight years
later, I am smiling still, in my ICU hospital bed, as I recall the
final words of the inspiring children's book. I am attempting to
focus on my positive thinking—through all the obstacles, set-
backs, disappointments, pain, humility, and angst that have visited me throughout my checkered life, and especially now. I am
calling on my basic optimism and positivity and feistiness and
competitive nature and the fighter in me to be strong and to
begin to heal.

I am thinking about self-confidence and how I survived everything I just endured. In my fog, I am considering the critical lexical difference between "I thought I could" and "I *knew*
I could." In the face of danger and doom, why should we
embrace tentative optimism instead of a healthy dose of committed self-belief? And I rewrite, with all due respect to Watty
Piper (actually, the pseudonym of publisher Arnold Munk), the
ending of *The Little Engine That Could* to better suit me, optimis-
tically and cardiologically speaking:

And the Little New Engine smiled and seemed to say as he
puffed steadily down the mountain. "I knew I could. I knew I
could. I knew I could. I knew I could.
I knew I could.
I knew I could.

As I recompose the ending of the story, it occurs to me that, as always, life is not so simple. And there's always the other side of the coin, or, rather, the other sides.

So then, was it really that: "I knew I could"? Well, maybe it was actually: "I was pretty darn sure I could." Or, more accurately: "I think I knew I could." Or even (here comes that guy Montaigne again): "What do I know?"

Which brings up, as I begin to regain a modicum of lucidity, the conundrum of faith and trust, one of the great dilemmas in the life of my mind. Ultimately, in what or whom do I put my faith? What or whom can I trust? God? The cosmic tumblers? Some other "higher force" outside of myself? The way things are meant to be? Something else? Nothing else? Other people? Myself? Or maybe a combo sandwich?

As I lie in bed, eyes closed and connected to life by my tubes and needles and catheters and monitors and medications, I am wondering what or who was responsible (beyond the control, that is, of the obvious answers: the cardiologists, the surgeon and his team, Susan) for my survival, in what or whom I had put my faith, making it possible for me to pull through. I am reflecting, in my now-dissipating fog, how for me, trust is a bit of an ironic concept: I am pretty much a right-brain type of person and consider myself a creative spirit who depends largely on instinct and intuition, yet to have trust in someone or something requires not only a gut feeling inside of me, but also the "uncreative" elements of experience and empiricism. I need to base my trust on what has worked before and what has been proven to me and to my satisfaction. I need results and consistency and dependability. I need for it *to be earned*. And thus far, what and whom I trust in my life are my own instincts (which have proven to be pretty darn dependable) and my wife and my family and my true friends. In this way, I guess I am an agnostic, in the literal sense: *I don't know* (that is, until I know).

My mind wanders to the story of Isaac, in Genesis 22, which, ever since Hebrew school nearly sixty years ago and through the years of being a father myself and up to the present, has always fascinated yet puzzled me, this story of pure faith in God (or the fear of Him, as the angel of the Lord describes it). Basically, God commands Abraham to sacrifice his only son, Isaac, as a burnt offering to Him. Abraham, unwavering in his obedience, binds Isaac and lays him on the altar and raises a knife to slay his only son. In the nick of time (but of course!), the angel of the Lord calls out from heaven and tells Abraham not to commit the deed. Instead, he sacrifices a ram instead of his son, and Isaac is spared! (I always wondered about the ram's loved ones, but that's another story for another book.)

Now we all know that this is a story, a parable, a metaphor. A lovely one at that, and one that defines as clear as a temple bell the meaning of pure and absolute loyalty. Or blind faith, if you will. But it is nonetheless a metaphor, and, in reality, no one in his or her right mind would ever take this story literally and act on it and slay an only child. Or, for that matter, believe that an obese, bearded man can fit into a chimney (bearing his fat bag of goodies, no less), slide down it (and in transit avoid all the soot), and deposit gifts in stockings for all the kiddies on the planet via his flying, reindeer-motored sleigh. In real life, for me anyway, I need something more concrete than that to merit my trust.

And speaking of only sons, I am recalling a story that demonstrates how very difficult it is to have *total and complete* faith in a "higher" power.

A thirtysomething Jewish mother is walking on a Long Island beach just behind her only child, her darling two-year-old son. Without warning: a deafening clap of thunder followed by a blinding bolt of lightning, and then an enormous tidal wave that reaches the shore, engulfing the little boy and sweeping him out to sea, presumably lost forever.

The mother is shocked, horrified, bereft, disconsolate, devastated.

In her grief, she looks up to the heavens in a desperate effort to negotiate with the Almighty.

"My Lord, *Melech ha'olom*, King of the universe, please, I beseech you, bring back my son!"

Panicking more by the second and hearing no response whatsoever, she continues her frantic plea, a torrent of tears now streaming down her trembling cheeks.

"Listen to me, God of my fathers, merciful and gracious Lord, please, I beg of you, bring back my son! I promise to you here and now that I will worship you every minute of every day until my last dying breath on Earth. I will consecrate my life to you, I will go to shul three times a week, I will read the Bible every day, I will be the best Jew and the best person I can possibly be. If you would only return to me my only child, my beloved Joshua."

With that, the mother hears a second tremendous clap of thunder and witnesses a second fearsome bolt of lightning, and then a second massive tidal wave crashes on the shore and deposits, no more than a foot in front of her and at her feet, her adorable Joshua. It is truly a miracle!

The mother is in awe upon spying her son, who is standing right there before her very eyes. Collecting herself, she stares at the boy for a moment, then gazes up at the heavens and says to the Almighty, in her most contentious New York Jewish accent, "He had a *hat?*"

I am still grappling with the questions of faith and trust, and with the way the world works. And how in the world I just got to where I am now.

Did I know, or did I think I knew, that things would work out well because of something *inside of me?* Probably. As a student, long ago, I was struck (and still am) by Ralph Waldo Emerson's statement in his profoundly wise essay "Self-reliance": "Trust thyself; every heart vibrates to that iron string."

Every . . . *heart.*

Before and after my transplant surgery, and over the course of the past three months, I have had many long chats with cardiologists, surgeons, and other physicians about the importance of attitude and self-belief and self-trust. They all tell me that, yes, it really helps that my body is strong for a seventy-year-old. (At my age, it isn't a given that I'd make it through the long surgery.) And yes, that being here at Cedars-Sinai is certainly a sine qua non, since very few hospitals anywhere would have accepted me as a heart transplant candidate at my age. But, most of all, that—as "unscientific" as it sounds—my having a positive attitude, inner strength, belief and trust in myself, and the determination and motivation to survive is quite possibly the most important factor of all. And I believe them, totally.

So, in the end, aside from my cardiologists and surgeons and Susan, of course, I relied on, well, *me*.

And that, as Robert Frost said at the end of "The Road Not Taken," has made all the difference.

I am now recalling having read somewhere that although the weight of the average Thoroughbred horse's heart is eight pounds or so, that of Secretariat—arguably the greatest race-horse ever, along with the equally awesome Man o' War—weighed in at autopsy at a whopping twenty-two pounds! And I am thinking about this physical advantage he had (stronger pumping mechanism, higher ejection fraction, more oxygen provided, etc.), but, at the same time, about the fact that he had a huge "inner" heart that stoked his unparalleled determination and drive to win. And I am thinking what a perfect metaphor that is of my situation, where I didn't possess a big or strong or healthy physical heart, but what helped me survive was my big "metaphysical" or spiritual heart, my drive and motivation to fight through all of this.

I am a spiritual person in some ways, but not in the formally religious sense. I believe that there may well be a higher power somewhere in the universe, or at least some sort of natural order, that is virtually unknowable and deeply personal. Of course, many people often feel the need to lean on or look to something greater than themselves. For them, God is a concept, a myth they need to believe in order to insert order in their lives and to be there when they need Him (or Her). Which is fine, with me and for them. In my experience, which has been marked by frequent challenges and sleeping policemen just like everyone else's—physical, moral, psychological, and emotional—I have personally chosen to rely for the most part on my own powers of resiliency and strength to overcome these challenges, failing often, succeeding occasionally. This intuition comes from deep inside of me and is spiritual in its own way. But that's my own take on the universe. I'm a very proactive person and always prefer to take matters into my own hands, when I can (these three last words being the obviously operative ones).

Take matters into my own hands. This phrase is evoking in me a reflection on *La Main de Dieu* (*The Hand of God*), Rodin's magnificent sculpture upon which my eyes first gazed back in the early seventies, in his eponymous museum in Paris.

A graduate student, I am transfixed by this amazing vertical white hand of God emerging from a rough, unfinished mass of marble as its base and wondering how Rodin ever got this massive hand to look so strong and yet so loving. I am staring at the back of the sculpture, at the back of God's hand extruding smooth and gentle and yet powerful from the mass of rough marble, and wondering how Rodin ever accomplished that. I am looking at the front of the statue, at Adam and Eve in a loving caress, he in her lap and cradling her head with his hands and their lips meeting tenderly and all the while the loving, miniature couple is being cradled themselves in this amazing, oversize hand of their awesome Creator (in both senses: God and Rodin the artist). I am wondering how the artist was ever able to make such a sensuous scene so innocent and glorious.

I am looking at the whole piece, at what a magnificent and sacred statement is being made from so few elements, how the very birth of humankind and of love on Earth could possibly have been expressed so simply and majestically by the sculpting of a single hand and the two vest-pocket creatures cradled by it and in it. I am looking for yet a ninth time at the awesome divine hand and the embracing bodies within, and I suddenly understand really and truly what a metaphor is and how powerful it can be when it simplifies and clarifies and concretizes something extremely abstract and otherwise nearly unfathomable.

Back in the present and my hospital bed, my eyes still closed, I am making the logical linguistic connection with the American spiritual "He's Got the Whole World in His Hands": a nice metaphor, as well, but here in the hospital and in dire need of a new heart and a second chance, the only hands I have had at my disposal—aside from the surgeons' and the nurses' and Susan's, of course—are mine. God's hand is a powerful metaphor, whether in Rodin's statue or in the song, but cruel reality is another thing, and during my crisis, I have needed the strength of something real that I could trust, and that something was me.

When it came down to it, I knew *in my heart* that I'd be okay. Or in my gut, if you prefer. My always-reliable compass—whether emotional, creative, or anything else—is my instinct, my intuition, my little voice inside, my Emersonian "iron string." A compass on which I have depended for my entire life, but especially during this hospital visit, when it came to the rescue countless times to give me hope and confidence. *Gnothi seauton!* These past three months have forced me to *know myself* way better than ever.

With a silly smile on my face, I am thinking of Shel Silverstein. I love Shel's poetry, his wise and profound and funny

musings. And at this particular moment, I am thinking of his
fitting piece "The Voice":

There is a voice inside of you
That whispers all day long,
"I feel that this is right for me,
I know that this is wrong."
No teacher, preacher, parent, friend
Or wise man can decide
What's right for you—just listen to
The voice that speaks inside.

I am revisiting a placard hanging in the soccer locker room
at Williams, a sign I looked at and was inspired by every time
I prepared for and recovered from soccer practices and games
when I was an undergrad. It said, simply: WHEN THE GOING
GETS TOUGH, THE TOUGH GET GOING.

Since my formative years, I guess I've always tended toward
self-based belief. Call it existentialist or transcendentalist or
Emersonian or whatever: in the end, you are the single entity
you know the best, and by far, so if you can't have faith in or
trust yourself, then . . .

On the other hand, maybe some form of God exists. Maybe,
to paraphrase 1988 vice presidential hopeful Senator Lloyd Bent-
sen, "Bob Mitchell, you're no Abraham." And maybe there is luck
and fate and destiny, too. And maybe things were meant to be.

What do I know?

I am dredging up from the past a quote from Blaise Pascal, one that I have loved forever: "*Le coeur a ses raisons, que la*

raison ne connaît point," "The heart has its reasons that reason doesn't have a clue about." Had "reason" or logic prevailed, any of the five VT episodes should have killed me. In my three-month battle against time, reason should have dictated that my old, sick heart give out before they found a new one for me. When they found the cancer, reason might have deduced that, undetected, it should have spread. When I entered the hospital, reason should have prevented me from becoming a candidate for the transplant in the first place. And when I entered the OR, at my age, for the actual transplant surgeries, reason should have determined that I not exit the room alive. No, the heart prevailed, both physically and figuratively, because it has its own "reasons." The great irony: Pascal's quote was meant to be a religious affirmation of faith, back in seventeenth-century France. My (lay) interpretation of his *coeur,* his "heart," is admittedly different from his, yet I cherish the fact that it is.

Funny, but I have written about this quotation from Pascal in academic papers, a collection of my poetry, and a few of my novels. But until now, it was a literary motif to me, an abstract—albeit lovely—concept. And now, in Cedars-Sinai Medical Center in Los Angeles, CA, I am actually—and miraculously—*living it.*

I open my eyes slowly, and Susan, my heroine, is by my side. She tells me that I have been out of it for hours since the surgery, mumbling to myself and making silly faces, and that I probably have no recollection of even being awake after the transplant surgery until now. She tells me that I have been groggy, my speech has been slurred, I have barely seemed to recognize her, and I have been falling in and out of sleep.

I am now relatively lucid, and I realize what has just happened. I can't believe that I survived the surgery, but: *I knew I could!*

Awakened finally from my deep daydream, I am, truly for the first time, realizing what has actually happened. Susan and I look deeply into each other's eyes. I feel like crying, laughing, screaming for joy, and getting down on my figurative knees in gratitude toward my generous donor and his generous family, my heart and kidney surgeons (Alfredo Trento and Irene Kim), the surgical teams, the entire medical and nursing staff at Cedars-Sinai, my strong supporter from Scripps (Ajay Srivastava), my kids and family and friends for their loving support, and, last but certainly not least, Susan herself. But in addition to and possibly above all these emotions, I am feeling a profound relief, that I made it and that I am here, living and breathing, and totally psyched to enter the game again (in centerfield, natch).

I'm certain that Susan is feeling the same emotions. Right now, we are neither crying nor laughing; instead, we both have these incredulous looks on our faces, in awe of what has happened, in awe of the medical technology and surgical skill from which I have benefited, in awe of the fact that, for whatever reason or reasons, *I am here.*

We spend the next couple of hours smiling, talking, hugging, reveling in a cocoon of joy, disbelief, and gratitude. At the end of which I am feeling beat and beat up, and we say our tender good-byes an instant before I crash.

When I awaken hours later, I am sad not to see Susan here by my bedside to comfort me. (She is my rod and my staff.)

The worst is over now, I hope and believe; and, after three days in the ICU, I am recovering in my new room, the proud owner of a twenty-nine-year-old heart and not one, not two, but two-and-a-half kidneys! A Swan-Ganz catheter, protruding from my jugular vein, is attached to a monitor. (Translation: I am not allowed to leave the room for the next I-don't-know-how-many days, when I will be discharged, once and hopefully for all, from Cedars-Sinai.)

I am noticing that I am having a great deal of trouble holding onto objects. I have abandoned my natural inclination to refuse help, now that I am helpless to do even the simplest of things: holding a cup or a pen or an eating utensil. I am now accepting aid, because I am getting tired of dropping and spilling food and drink all over my bed and gown. And I need the nurses or Susan to write down notes for me (for my writing or for stray thoughts or to fill in the daily menu orders), because my hands are shaking uncontrollably from the surgery and all the immunosuppressants and steroids (mostly the prednisone) I'm on now. I can barely hold a pen (how humiliating for a writer!), and my penmanship is on sabbatical: whenever I try to scribble something down, it looks nearly as illegible as a physician's handwriting on a prescription form. Happily, one thing I *can* hold onto, and firmly, is hope.

On the second day after the surgery, before Susan's imminent visit, I am thinking about a subject that has come up so often during my stay at Cedars-Sinai, not to mention all of my life: luck, randomness, and the meaning of it all. I am feeling sorrow and empathy for the unfortunate young man who was killed in the accident. And, of course, for his family and friends. Yet, so very ironically, I am also thinking of how fortuitous (lucky?) it was that he perished at that very moment, just in time for my life to be saved. Am I being selfish? Opportunistic? Perhaps. But at the same time, the feelings of gratitude and relief are just as powerful. And the solace of believing that the grieving family of the deceased donor is, I am guessing, comforted in the knowledge that their loved one's heart and kidney are helping someone in desperate shape to survive.

Alone, I am staring at my battered body. My hands and arms, riddled with plum-colored blotches (hematomas from the hefty doses of prednisone, a corticosteroid and an immunosuppressant), give me the appearance of a spotted hyena. I am staring at the eight-inch-long chest incision; the five-and-a-half-inch-long kidney incision; the seven perforation scars from the nephrectomy; the twenty-nine-year-old (the exact same age as my new heart!), two-foot-long, bypass-surgery, saphenous vein scar from my left groin to my left ankle; the two defibrillator surgery scars (my device was removed during the transplant surgery). I am concentration-camp skinny, my formerly powerful and muscular legs are unrecognizably atrophied, and—as a special, surprise bonus—my feet are bloated from gout.

The image of one of Andrea Mantegna's paintings of the martyr St. Sebastian appears before my eyes (next time you're in the Kunsthistorisches Museum in Vienna, check it out: I'm sure it's on your bucket list). The thirteen—unlucky?—arrows stuck in his body (one going into his jugular and out his forehead, one into his heart, one into his right kidney!). The blood. His calm, saintly gaze toward the heavens. How does he manage this? It doesn't look human (he's a saint, after all). I feel his pain, if not his peace of mind.

But right now, I don't really give a rat's ass about how I look. I made it through all of this, and the rest is not silence, as Hamlet said at the end, but . . . *tiny potatoes.*

On the other hand (the concepts of ullage, syzygy, paradox, and the two sides of the coin again ring true!) . . .

Ah, senescence. Looking at how I have changed physically, I can't help thinking—for the first time in a truly serious way— about the potentially depressing process of growing old. Perhaps because I am aware of the toll the surgery and lead-up have taken on my physical body, to ponder this concept now seems an obvious consequence.

My mind now turns, morbidly and naturally, toward death. Huh? A seventy-plus-year-old man who just had double-transplant surgery thinking about getting old and facing death? What a shock! On the other hand, I may look like an old man right now, but I don't feel like one inside. On the other hand (at the risk of sounding like *Fiddler on the Roof*'s Tevye), I was just running around like a dervish with my Spaldeen, and look at me now.

A stupid smile creases my face as my mind conjures up images of movie actors from the forties: Barry Fitzgerald, James Gleason, Edward G. Robinson, Henry Travers, Charles Bickford, Frank Morgan, Charles Coburn, S. Z. Sakall, Thomas Mitchell, George Sanders, Walter Brennan, Claude Rains, Sidney Greenstreet, Walter Huston, William Demarest, Monty Woolley. I chortle internally: and I think *I* look old?

Funny thing is, whenever I saw these "old-timers" in films of yore—as a kid or even recently—I always thought they looked pretty dang old, weather-beaten even, maybe in their seventies or even eighties. While in reality, they were probably only in their fifties. What pity, even Schadenfreude, I felt for those old geezers! How very close to death they always seemed! This thought picks up my spirits a bit, because even now, a shell of my former self, I look a lot younger than all of them, in my humble—and humbled—opinion.

My frozen smile remains as I picture my younger daughter, Sarah, handing me a birthday gift when she was ten maybe and I was in my midforties. I open (tear off) the wrapping, and inside is a black T-shirt with sparkly, colored letters that spell out: OLDER THAN DIRT.

Now, even with all my surgical battle wounds and my gauntness and my skeletal appearance, I am definitely feeling younger than dirt. *Way* younger.

To celebrate my survival (at my relatively advanced age), I sing to myself—attempting to employ Paul Robeson's inimitable bass-baritone voice, of course—the iconic aria written by Oscar Hammerstein II, from the musical *Showboat*:

> *Ol' man river, dat ol' man river*
> *He mus' know sumpin', but don't say nuthin'*
> *He jes' keeps rollin'*
> *He keeps on rollin' along*

Now Edgar Allan Poe effortlessly surfaces in my consciousness. He was the first "real" writer of which I became conscious during my formative years (followed shortly by Dickens and Dostoevsky). I think I was in sixth grade. Classmate Ray Rizzuti turned me on to him, and I immediately read most of Poe's short stories. I became obsessed with his writing, especially the first short story of his that I read, "The Tell-Tale Heart."

Briefly, the narrator of the story carefully plans the murder of an old man, commits it, dismembers the body, and hides the pieces under the floorboards of the old man's room. The police arrive, sit in chairs, and suspect nothing. The narrator, frantically imagining that he hears the violent beating of the old man's heart from under the floorboards, finally confesses to the crime:

> *"Villains!" I shrieked, "dissemble no more! I admit the deed! —tear up the planks! here, here!—It is the beating of his hideous heart!"*

I am pondering this story because my own heart—my old man's new and beautiful, not hideous, heart—somehow refuses to stop beating and lives on!

I am lying on my left side, just lying here peacefully, and something absolutely astounding occurs to me. I am suddenly aware of the fact that since my defibrillator—which corrected the damaged electrical circuitry of my old heart—was removed during the surgery, 1. I don't have that protruding box in my upper left chest anymore; 2. because its wires used to lean against my phrenic nerve, causing my heart to beat violently whenever I lay on my left side, this pounding has obviously disappeared (the traumatic thumping not only made it really difficult to fall asleep, but it made me feel like that old Looney Tunes Sylvester the Cat cartoon, where Sylvester has just fallen in love, and his pounding cartoon heart—*boing boing!*—is literally leaping out of his chest, attached to his body by this Slinky-looking springy thing); and 3. lo and behold: now, defibrillatorless, I can finally sleep on my left side, without losing my sanity . . . *for the rest of my life!*

These thoughts about the mechanical nature of the heart, and all its electrical qualities, incite another heated discussion with my inner self. We humans are, of course, all sentient beings. We have feelings, often complex ones. (This is the Romantic part of me.) But, I ask myself, why have we—in most civilizations and since Biblical days—always ascribed the cause of emotions and feelings to *the heart*? Because it beats more quickly when we are in an emotional state, whether it is fear, love, pain, passion, or anger? On the other hand, the heart is just an electric pump, right? (This is the Realist part of me.) In point of fact, and if you insist on getting technical, it's actually the brain that gives it orders to beat faster. Scientifically speaking, it is the brain—and specifically the amygdala and the medulla oblongata—that processes emotions, then gives its marching orders to the heart to beat faster, which the heart does, as an obedient foot soldier—or, rather, chest soldier. So why not ascribe feelings and emotions to their true source, *the brain*? Shouldn't we really be saying, "I love you from the bottom of my brain" and "Be still, my brain" and "I am sending my brainfelt condolences" and even (dare I say it?) "time for a brain-to-brain"?

And then it suddenly hits me, *and hard*: I have a brand new heart, right here in my chest, right where my old, sick, dying heart I've had for seventy years used to be! I have the heart of a twenty-nine-year-old. A heart that will transform my life completely and allow me to have all the physical energy and stamina to live a normal, healthy life and to accomplish all my unfinished business, and then some. How amazing it is to have had this procedure just in the nick of time, before my old heart gave in. And, to boot, to have dodged the cancer bullet. *Holy kamoley!*

I am shaken out of my reverie by the ringing of my cell phone ("Centerfield"). It is a thoughtful and caring call from my old—and I mean old!—friend, Hank Gardstein, whom I've now known for sixty-one years. We were pals starting in fifth grade, in 1954, then through high school, when he met his future wife, Elayne, at a party in my Brooklyn basement. And we've remained great pals to this day. (Hank and Elayne are still married, and Susan and I consider them among our very dearest friends.) Then, soon after, I receive loving calls from my three kids (Noah, Jenny, Sarah), which activated my amygdala and medulla oblongata and which made my new heart feel *real* good. And then a wonderful Skype session with our dear Roman friends, Giuseppe Signorile and Maria Gravina. Then, during the next few hours, ten more phone calls from other close friends. (Without mentioning names: my dear aunt Phyllis, Frank and Barbara Fleizach, Mary and Lance Donaldson-Evans, Mike Appelbaum, Pete and Linda Haller, Stan and Carroll Possick, Kenny and Paula Horn, Val Light and Bob Joseph, Anthony Caprio, Bill and Beth Jaquith.) And a bunch of e-mails from other dear friends. (Without mentioning names: Leo and Margaret Schwartz, Judith Bluysen, Mark Cripps, Tania Calcinaro and Marco Croci, Meredith Geisler, Rony and Rachel Herz, Mauro Cazzaro and Antonella Maione, David and Joanne Frantz, Seymon and Lynne Ostilly, Suzanne Nash, the Finkelstein cousins Lee, Ellen, Steven, and Eric.)

I am filled with hope for the future and for my survival. It's good to be loved. I have so much to live for!

And then, icing on the cake, my guardian angel, Susan, enters the room, fresh from her two-hour drive from Carlsbad. As usual, she brings into my hospital room yearned-for and much-appreciated rays of sunshine. A Robert Frost quote instantly comes to mind as she closes the door behind her:

> *Then all I need do is run*
> *To the other end of the slope*
> *And to tracts laid new to the sun,*
> *Begin all over to hope.*

A few hours after Susan arrives, a(nother) breath of fresh air, this time by the name of Dr. Michelle Kittleson, enters my room. Her name—as the cardiologist in charge of my case—has been on my parakeet-like wristband for nearly three months now, yet this is the first time we have ever met face-to-face. Michelle is a very bright, very upbeat, very encouraging, very energetic, and very ebullient person, a rare combo for a doctor, at least in my experience. Best of all, she is a wonderful teacher, answering all my cardiological questions clearly, decisively, and without a trace of dumbing down or condescension. And a wonderful listener, to boot. But what distinguishes her in this (understandably) rigid hospital environment is her flexibility, empathy, and iconoclastic streak when it comes to confronting the morass of draconian rules.

After a few minutes of getting to know each other:

"So, Michelle, the nurses are telling me that a bunch of foods are now forbidden to me. Can you help me out on this?"

"Which ones concern you the most?" she answers caringly.

"Well, I guess I can live without grapefruit, because I understand clearly about the contraindications with new meds. Same thing for sushi and fried eggs, with the risk of bacteria. But what about red meat? I mean, a good medium-rare steak or burger . . . I'm not so sure I can give those things up forever. I know about the risk of bacteria with meat cooked below medium, but *really!*"

"Well," Michelle begins with a kindly smile, "I *am* concerned about rejection—"

"I am, too, believe me! But after getting this second chance, I dunno. On the one hand, I don't want to risk any rejection, but on the other, I need to live my life, or what remains of it, with joy and pleasure!"

"You know, Bob, you're exactly right. I couldn't agree more. Yes, don't go crazy or take big risks. But there's a happy medium you can reach, and if the risks are calculated, that's okay with me. So maybe somewhere between medium and medium-rare, but closer to medium, that would be fine."

"A happy . . . *medium?* I love it! Oh, and what about pizza? Once a month?" I ask, pseudotimidly.

"How about every other week?" Michelle replies with a conspiratorial wink.

"Great! And here's the biggie: I was told by someone, either a nurse or a doctor, that I can't consume alcohol anymore. Now, I've always enjoyed a single-malt Scotch every night before dinner, and I promise not to do that anymore. But how about, say, if I pour myself a short drink, two fingers maybe, oh, once a week or so?"

I await nervously while Michelle spends a quality two seconds cogitating and deciding my fate.

"Deal!" she says.

I think I love you, I whisper silently.

At the risk of pushing my luck with her, I continue my pleading. "Do I have to wear a mask in a restaurant, if we go early, say, at 5:30?"

"Nope."

"And one of the nurses told us that I shouldn't cross my legs!" I follow. "Something about circulation problems. Does that sound right to you?"

Michelle tilts her head slightly to her left, like the dog Nipper in the old RCA Victor logo. "Of course you can cross your legs!" she says decisively. She is in my corner all the way, Angelo Dundee to my Ali. "In a nutshell, you know your body best. Just do everything in moderation, keep your fats and salt down, and you'll be just fine."

Her cheery optimism and compassion are just what the doctor ordered.

Three days later, I am alerted that this will be the day of my discharge from the hospital. I am armed to the teeth with twenty-six bottles of new medications, including immunosuppressants (to prevent my body from attacking my new heart), steroids, cholesterol suppressants, blood sugar suppressants, antibiotics, anti-infectives, antivirals, antidepressants, antacids, thyroid hormones, vitamins, aspirin, and channel blockers, to name a few; a blood sugar kit; and manuals, binders, folders, and detailed instructions about how to avoid infection, rejection, and death. Voluminous pages of what not to eat or drink (less-than-medium red meat, grapefruit, sushi, fried eggs over easy or medium, alcohol for at least three months), touch (people who sneeze, cough, or have health issues; babies; any surface that has been touched by living beings; doorknobs and the like; canine fecal matter), breathe in (air in close proximity to other humans), and do (intense exercise, walking on surfaces that might have broken glass that could cause me to bleed to death, run in a marathon, swim in a pool, be anywhere near a crowd, climb Mount Everest). Small potatoes in the scheme of things, because *I am outta here!* I am finally discharged after one hundred days in the various hospitals (including seventy-six at Cedars-Sinai). And after losing thirty-five pounds and enduring all the boredom, self-doubt, humility, pain, near-death bullets dodged, possibilities of rejection and infection, five CT and PET scans, four biopsies, three surgeries, two new organs, and a partridge in a you-know-what. Life is good. Life is *very* good.

I am sitting on my bed, waiting for Susan to arrive. I am, as usual, staring out my window, and as I gaze down at the concrete and the people walking on it, a white pigeon flaps its way across the window, then out of sight. I would not ordinarily notice this, but now I sure do. In a weird, Proustian way, my involuntary memory kicks into gear instantly, as the bird is recalling a meaningful and chilling moment, from about five years before, that has since haunted me and the deeper meaning of which has always been unclear to me. Until now.

I am walking our two Labs, Koslo and Mocha, in our Santa Barbara neighborhood. Just a few days before, my cardiologist,

Alan Brown, had mentioned to me that because of my arrhythmia issues, he might want me to go down to Cedars-Sinai in LA to have it checked out. My mind is preoccupied with going down there and possibly finding out that something is wrong, or abnormal, or even life-threatening. And then, smack in the middle of my lugubrious thoughts, I witness something that gives me a shudder that I can still feel to this day: a white pigeon plummeting down from the sky, from out of nowhere, with all the tragic suddenness of white-wingèd Icarus falling helplessly into the sea. The bird plummets vertically like a stone and crashes onto the ground on its back, right before my eyes. I stop and stare at the deceased pigeon and notice on its otherwise pristine breast a perfectly round, one-inch-in-diameter, bright crimson stain. Either someone shot it (no way!) or . . . or . . . it died suddenly of a massive myocardial infarction! Was this a sign (I don't particularly believe in them)? Was it an omen (ditto)? I was pretty freaked out at the time because of my own precarious heart history. But now, as I await my departure from Cedars-Sinai, and having successfully survived my heart ordeal, the pigeon of my past is no longer the Pigeon of Doom; it has become the Pigeon of Hope. Sadly, I am thinking, some don't make it through their heart ordeals. But some, like me, do.

A game of inches.

And now, the time has finally come to vacate the premises and restart my life. I place myself in a wheelchair for the final time—I proudly refuse a nurse's kind offer to help—and, with my amazing Susan by my side, am rolled down the hall to the elevator. We descend to the ground floor of the Tower. And here we are at the Exit Door. My mind wanders to Canto III, line

9, of Dante's *Inferno,* the passage with the quote inscribed on the Entrance Gate of Hell: "*Lasciate ogni speranza, voi ch'entrate,*" "Abandon all hope, ye who enter here." How true this must seem to so many patients entering this place with life-threatening conditions, including those waiting for a new heart! But here I am, making my exit, finally, having vanquished a long list of obstacles and especially that nefarious villain, hopelessness. And despite all the incredible care and gifts that Cedars-Sinai has bestowed upon me, I can't help feeling a visceral sense of unadulterated relief in departing. A divine smile etched on my gaunt face and with hope filling my heart, I exit the hospital, joyously, for the last time as an inpatient.

11
Next!

Roseanne Roseannadanna, that great philosopher, said it best: "Well, it just goes to show you, it's always something—if it ain't one thing, it's another."

What wisdom is hidden in these seemingly vacuous and meaningless words! What a fine line between apparent nonsense and profound sagacity! Yes, there are no absolutes in life. Happiness, misery, wealth, poverty, well-being, infirmity? They all change and fluctuate and appear and reappear cyclically, because, in fact, it *is* always something! That's what makes life fascinating, having the pendulum going back and forth, sempiternally.

And that "something" that Roseanne is talking about is usually something bad, or at least unexpected, and almost always both. Since my discharge from Cedars-Sinai, I have been thinking a lot about *my* recent somethings: the VT attacks, then the hospitals, then the IV drips, then the LVAD scare, then the change of strategy to the transplant, then the waiting list and the waiting, then more IV drips, then all those tests and scans and ultrasounds and biopsies, then the cancer, then the cancer surgery, then the recovery, then back on the list, then more waiting, then the transplant surgery, then the recovery . . .

If it ain't one thing, it's another.

Susan and I are now staying in a hotel room not far from the Hollywood Bowl (the hotel where Janis Joplin died tragically in 1970 from a heroin overdose) for one month, to be near Cedars-Sinai for my biweekly heart biopsies and clinics. We have to be moved from our first room because nothing works, the walls in our new room are a speck thicker than tissue paper and there is major construction (putting in floors) next door, there's a beastly heat wave going on in LA, and nocturnal bedspring sounds are emanating sporadically from above our ceiling, from what we surmise is a young couple not short on concupiscence. But, to be honest, Susan and I don't give a crap. We are here, living and breathing, and what might ordinarily bother us just rolls off our backs.

Time to think.

I am thinking about the one hundred days I have just spent on life-support IV drips in the four hospitals, about how the hospitals were a crucible, a huge personal test for me that produced lots of thought, much of which centered around the flaws I possess as a human being. In a sense, the hospitals were—aside from the places that saved my life—living, breathing metaphors, symbols of my weakness and fragility and vulnerability. In the hospital, my bodily flaws were obviously blatant, inside and out. But I also had all that time for my character to be tested (again), and to think about it, and the whys of it all, and what to do in the future. Lessons to be learned.

Not to say that we should all experience this elongated hospital wretchedness to do all that soul-searching. It's just that in our daily busy-ness, we generally don't have the time for such in-depth self-examination and rigorous testing. Maybe, in retrospect and in some vaguely twisted way, I'm actually thankful for having had this opportunity to learn some vital lessons, to make sense of it all (life, that is), to make proverbial lemonade out of proverbial lemons.

For some reason, my mind drifts to the dogs I have had in my life. God, how I love dogs! They are the best. Especially Mocha and Koslo, our two beloved Labs who have moved on to a better doggie life (although: how much better could it be there than down here?). Dogs bring out the best in us. They show us how simple life is, how uncomplicated love is, how easy it is to achieve unadulterated happiness. But, by contrast, they also show us how complicated our own lives are and how flawed we are as humans. Then again, they will never know the joys of listening to Beethoven, gazing at a Rodin sculpture, reading Dante or Shakespeare, rooting for their favorite team, hitting a winning backhand down the line or canning a serpentine twenty-foot putt, or even finishing the *New York Times* Sunday crossword puzzle in ink. So who would you rather be, if you had the choice, that is: Fido or you? (This is a trick question.)

So now that the gods have smiled upon me big-time and given me my Get-Out-of-Jail-Free card, I am at last beginning to enjoy life once again and to train my body to get back to normal. But wait a sec. Was it "the gods" who have smiled upon me? Funny I should use the term now, because in my gut, I feel that I was in the right place at the right time, that things just happened for the best, and mostly that my "luck" was influenced mightily by a powerful combination of various noncelestial factors: the extreme sickness of my heart; the support of the committees at both Scripps and Cedars-Sinai, who saw something in me that was worthy of being saved and being put on the 1A waiting list; the incredible competence and compassion of the medical teams at both Scripps and Cedars; my physical fitness (aside from my sick heart); the coincidence of my donor's car accident; my inner strength and grit and fighting spirit and positive attitude and determination to survive; and, of course, my motivation to live and not to give up my writing, my other passions, my friends and family, my children, and—the source of much of my strength and the major factor that made my survival possible—my Susan. All combining in concert and synergy to get me out of jail . . . free! Nah, I don't really think it was the smiling of the gods: *Luck is the residue of design.*

Our days are filled with joy, from dawn to dusk and beyond. Sure, there are frustrations, pesky side effects, loads of pain and discomfort, and obstacles (not to mention the annoyingly frequent heart biopsies), but by and large, we have zippo to complain about.

Our minds and bodies are occupied by good things: my PT rehab (I use a can of artichokes and one of black beans as weights for my improvised bicep curls), daily walks on a gorgeous Santa Monica beach, relishing nonhospital food, making plans for the future, just holding hands. Forget about the Roman poet Horace's "*Carpe diem.*" Our motto is now "*Carpe momentum,*" "Seize the moment"!

The bad news: my legs are still weak, and I have lots of pain moving around, getting in and out of bed, taking showers, and walking up steps, all the results of broken ribs and bruised chest muscles and incision scar pain from the surgeries. I must avoid sneezing at any cost, I walk up the steps to the hotel by holding onto the railing (not only am I too weak to do it on my own, but the broiling early September sun has turned the railing into a scorching furnace of molten steel), I am forced to endure the various side effects of my meds and the lengthy surgery: arms purple with hematomas, a propensity to bleed a lot and easily, headaches and dizziness, slightly thinning hair (which will repair itself eventually). The happy irony accompanying the latter affliction is that all these years through all my cardiac issues, I always told people that my dad had bequeathed to me a full head of hair and a bum ticker, and if I had my druthers, I'd opt to be bald and have a healthy heart. Well, now I am far from bald, but the thinning hair and the new heart are spookily realizing, yet happily disproving, my self-fulfilling prophecy of the idiom "Be careful what you wish for."

The great news: after a few weeks, I have developed an amazing appetite, I am sleeping much better (sometimes, admittedly, with the help of Ambien or Benadryl), I have way more strength and endurance, I am peeing way better (my new kidney!), and I can actually walk up staircases and steps without getting out of breath. And best news of all: *I am here!*

One beastly hot morning, Susan and I are driving from our room to the hospital for my clinic and heart biopsy. Every little sleeping policeman in the street is a major challenge for my tender and vulnerable chest muscles and ribs. As we stop at a red light, I notice, to my right, a guy—who sort of looks like me and is about my age—limping along La Cienega Blvd., bedraggled, hunched over (as if by the enormous weight of the world and all his worries), homeless perhaps, sporting a longish gray beard and jeans as tired-looking as he. This poor wretch, I am thinking, could well be kind, giving, talented, and brilliant. He could be fully capable of contributing a great deal to the world and of helping and giving love to others. *What do I know?* I am thinking: there but for the grace of God go I. Or, maybe more aptly for me: there but for the grace of someone or something out there or dumb luck or chance or destiny or fate or outside forces or circumstances or an inch here or there or whatever . . . go I.

One night, after dinner, and after all I've just been through, I am seriously pondering a wise, wonderful quote bequeathed to me thirty years ago by a dear old friend from my advertising days, Frank Fleizach (you may remember him as my inspiration for "The Torre Story" way back in Chapter 2). It is a one-word, four-letter quote about the paradoxical and unpredictable nature of life that is pithy, practical, and profound and that I have never forgotten:

"Next!"

So, my plans didn't exactly pan out? So, life, what *else* do you have to throw at me? *Huh?* And once again, all the ups and downs of my life flash before me.

Okay, so I work really hard in high school and earn a BA, an MA, and a PhD and teach at Harvard, Purdue, and Ohio State and publish four books on French poetry and throw myself totally into my teaching. Life is good. Then, out of nowhere, my ex-wife doesn't want to live in Ohio anymore. *Next!*

Okay, so I pick myself up, move my family to New York, start a new career in advertising as a junior copywriter at the ripe old age of thirty-seven, work my way up to creative director, win lots of awards, shoot commercials all over the world. Life is good. Then, out of nowhere, I have a massive heart attack, losing twenty-five percent of my heart muscle, and have quadruple-bypass surgery. *Next!*

Okay, so I pick myself up, win more awards, keep shooting spots all over the world, and my kids are growing up nicely. Life is good. Then, out of nowhere, comes a very bad year in the business, and I am canned. I am unemployed, with two kids in college and one not too far behind. *Next!*

Okay, so I pick myself up, land a great gig in Tel Aviv teaching commercial film writing and production (an experience of a lifetime, even though I have to do it alone and away from my family), make enough to support my family for a year. Life is good. Then, out of nowhere, my ex-wife rings me up from the States at 2 a.m. one fine morning to ask for a divorce after twenty-seven years of marriage. *Next!*

Okay, so I pick myself up, pack up my stuff and my guitars and my tennis racquets, and move to California. I am writing nonfiction books on sports and giving tennis lessons, to make ends meet, and I love it. Life is good. Then, out of nowhere, I have a second heart attack, an angioplasty, and, just as a little bonus, a defibrillator inserted inside my chest. *Next!*

Okay, so I pick myself up, recover, spend a year living in Paris, Stockholm, London, and Tel Aviv trying to figure out what I will do in life, and where in the world I will live. Life is good. Then, out of nowhere, I have an epiphany: I will, as I have always longed to do, start all over and write novels. *Next!*

Okay, so I pick myself up, move to beautiful Santa Barbara, fall in love with and marry a wonderful woman (Susan), write four novels, adore what I do and where I live. And to top it off, my three kids are now independent and thriving. Life is good. Then, out of nowhere, I have another heart attack and surgery, our two beloved Labrador Retrievers die, and we can't afford to live in Santa Barbara anymore. *Next!*

Okay, so we pick ourselves up, move to beautiful Carlsbad, and plan to live there happily ever after. Life is *very* good. Then, out of nowhere, I have my five V-tach attacks, spend one hundred days in hospitals on IV life support, and endure cancer surgery and heart and kidney transplants . . .

You get the picture.

12
Life is Goo!

Dante wasn't the only one to make the journey from hell to paradise, I muse as I gaze upon a perfect, sun-and-cumulus-filled Southern California sky from a comfy chaise longue on our patio in Carlsbad. Like the great Florentine poet, I have emerged from the shadows of the underworld and arrived at a place of ecstasy, struggling throughout my extraordinary journey from hell and purgatory to paradise. And guided all the while, nobly and wisely, not by Virgil (as was Dante), but by Susan.

It is September 6, 2015, forty-one days after my double-transplant surgery. Here I am, miraculously, back in the saddle, alive and kicking. And home at last.

Look at me, I can be centerfield!

In my lifetime, I have lived in many different places—in seven states in the US and in Canada, Israel, France, the UK, Italy, and Sweden. Each location was just right for me at that precise time in my life. Whether it was growing up or spending my summers or doing research or writing books or teaching or raising a family or starting an ad agency or looking for employment or finding myself or for sheer pleasure and adventure.

And now I am in Carlsbad, CA, at a time of my life where tranquillity and ideal weather and proximity to the ocean are absolute sine qua nons to my happiness and productivity. I constantly find the beaches, ocean, and hills (here, they remind me of parts of Umbria or Tuscany) to be soothing and reassuring. I find that where I have now landed for the duration, after all my stops along the way, is the perfect place to give me the space and time to think and write and rehab and return to normalcy and peace and contentment. And now—particularly under the circumstances and in the perspective of my recent adventure—it is, of all the great places I've ever lived in, the greatest.

A few days after we are here, Susan and I take our first walk in eons on one of our beautiful local beaches. It is, as Dante would say, *il paradiso.* As we walk, we listen to the sounds of the waves lapping against the shore. We watch birds gliding and swooping, and scooting on the sand: seagulls, pelicans, marbled godwits, whimbrels, plovers, cormorants. We are accompanied, in the background, by surfers and paragliders and the occasional walker or jogger, yet we are utterly alone. We are holding hands and hunting casually for heart rocks and talking giddily about everything and nothing.

And just being outdoors! As I walk the beach, I recall so vividly looking sadly and frequently out of my hospital room window in LA at the people down there living their lives, free as plovers to walk around and breathe the fresh (albeit smoggy) air. And now, here I am, walking on a beach and inhaling deeply the fresh, breezy, delicious ocean air. Many of us probably take this simple phenomenon of being outdoors for granted. But not if you've been penned up in a hospital room for over three months. Just think about it. I do, and nonstop.

A quote by Thoreau glides effortlessly into my brain: "Sometimes as I drift on Walden Pond, I cease to exist and begin to be." It's sure good to be alive, but it's even better to be *living*.

How grateful I am! First, for just being here. For the care and competence of my docs at Scripps and Cedars-Sinai. For the enormous generosity of my donor and his family. For the love and support of my family and friends. And last but not least, for Susan's fortitude and grit and positive thoughts and undying love, which I am absolutely certain helped save my life every bit as much as the surgery did.

Speaking of which.

I am ambivalent—sometimes skeptical, sometimes a true believer—regarding the sentimental concept of "this was meant to be." Maybe my surviving the whole heart (and kidney) thing was meant to be. Maybe my dodging the cancer bullet was meant to be. But then again—here comes the skepticism—if either of these crises had claimed my life, maybe that, too, would have been "meant to be." My good old friend *ullage* strikes again: the two equally viable sides of the coin of life.

I am beginning to conclude that for most things, maybe it isn't that they are meant to be or that they "happen for a reason." To turn the expression around, maybe the reason things happen is that they just happen, for that reason, which is, oddly, for no reason whatsoever. They just happen to us. Sometimes for better, sometimes for worse. I am coming to the conclusion that after living for seven decades on Earth, and having all of literature and philosophy at my disposal and all of my thinking about life to ponder in order to come up with some pithy and perfectly condensed aphorism for the meaning of life, maybe the best way to describe it is with these two frontal and innocent words: *Shit happens.* (Funny, because two-word maxims seem to appeal to me: *meden agan, gnothi seauton,* and, of course, "Less Miserable.") Yes indeed, shit does happen. Both good shit and bad shit and shit somewhere in between. It has and it does and it always will. For some reason or for no reason. Maybe what happens in the world is random after all, with no guiding force from outside of us. Maybe we just do our best and try our best and throw ourselves into the process of living and creating and doing good, and, in spite of and beyond us, the chips just fall where they may. Meanwhile, the constant and necessary ingredient for happiness and fulfillment, for me, is to continue to hope and believe in myself (and at times in chosen others) and to cherish the attributes of determination and motivation and strength and, of course, passion in the pursuit of everything.

Because of what has happened to my heart, I am constantly mulling over the concept of "this was meant to be." So *was* it?

Maybe it was or maybe it wasn't, but there is one thing in life I *am* certain was "meant to be," and that is my meeting Susan and discovering that we were soul mates for life. But why, you might ask, am I so sure of this?

For one thing, aside from the fact that we were attracted to each other from so many points of view, we discovered early on that we had this "Chuckles" thing going for us. You know, those multicolored jelly candies with the sugar coating. We both used to consume packs of Chuckles when we were kids (I in the fifties, she in the sixties). One evening, soon after we first met, she and I happened to be discussing candy of yore, and I pop the question.

"Remember Chuckles?"

"Yeparooney!" Susan answers. "They were great. Loved 'em!"

"Well, just for fun, let's name our favorite flavors, in ascending order worst to best, at the same time, at the count of three. Ready? One . . . two . . . three!"

"Green!" we shout out simultaneously.

"Okay, great. Now next, ready? One . . . two . . . three!"

"Yellow!" we exclaim concurrently.

"Hmm, this is getting interesting! Now next, ready? One . . . two . . . three!"

"Orange!" we blurt at the same time.

Our eyes meet in disbelief and pleasure.

"Okay. One . . . two . . . three!"

"Black!"

Now we know this was meant . . .

"One . . . two . . . three!"

. . . to . . .

"Red!"

. . . *be.*

"You cannot be *serious!*" I say with my most incredulous, guttural, McEnroesque inflection.

"Yep, this is a *definite* sign!" Susan opines emphatically.

And it was. But, you might protest, lots of couples share that very same order of Chuckles preferences. And you'd be correct (right off the bat, red is obviously the best, and green and yellow both suck big-time), so if it please the court, let me present as evidence the following follow-up "meant to be" corroborating anecdote.

When we make the decision to live together soon after we first met, Susan brings some of her "stuff" to the house I was renting in Santa Barbara (she had been living and working in her bungalow art studio closer to the ocean). As she is unpacking, she lifts out of one of her boxes one of her favorite pieces of art, a black-framed poster of the wonderful California street artist Robert Weil that she had acquired a few decades earlier. When I see it, my jaw drops.

"No *way!*" I roar, then race to my writing study, take a picture off the wall, bring it to Susan, and place it beside hers. My piece of art is one of my favorites, a black-framed poster of the wonderful California street artist Robert Weil that I had acquired a few decades earlier. When she sees it, her jaw drops.

Written on my poster is "Robert Weil Multiples/Robert Stein Fine Arts San Francisco." It is a wry, cartoonish print of a long, straight, skinny disembodied man's arm, covered by a gray jacket with white cuff and skinny hand protruding out of it, reaching out from the right edge of the poster (where it is cropped off at the elbow) and dispassionately pinching the nipple of a disembodied woman's breast, to the left. Written on Susan's poster is "Robert Weil/Recent Poster Works/Summer 1978." It is a wry, cartoonish print of a mustachioed man's head, covered by a bowler hat, peering out from the left edge of the poster (where it is cropped off at the chin) and dispassionately staring down at a naked woman's backside at the beach, to the right.

Can you imagine? What are the odds? A million to one? A quadrillion? To what can one attribute this unimaginable phenomenon? Two different people, in separate lives before coming together, purchasing, on separate coasts, posters by the same local California artist that had the very same wryly erotic motif, not identical in subject matter but eerily complementary, fitting each other like a matching pair, similar yet different, as if they were two pieces of a jigsaw puzzle just waiting to find each other and to be joined together perfectly? Was this coincidence? Serendipity? Synchronicity? Call it what you will, but for us, then and now, this moment screamed out, *"This was meant to be!"* Before then, and even now, I'm not sure I believe in this concept. Then again . . . *what do I know?*

From that moment on, the two prints have been proudly displayed on a special wall in our kitchen dedicated to them ("mine" on the left, "hers" on the right). It is our "Tits and Ass" wall (a tip of the bowler to Edward Kleban and Marvin Hamlisch for their cheeky song in *A Chorus Line*). It is very dear to us and reminds us, every day, of why we're spending our lives together on this planet.

Oh, how terribly wrong I was in that game of pennyball against Michael Krumholz sixty-two years ago! It has taken me this long, but I have finally seen the light and learned my (life) lesson:

DO-OVERS ARE INDEED PERMITTED HERE.

Susan and I return to our blessedly simple routine: beach walks, workouts in the gym, barbecuing on the patio, my writing and her art, keeping in touch with friends and family.

Getting back to my writing is especially satisfying for me. Throwing myself once again into one of my great passions (this time I am writing this memoir, about which I am particularly passionate), after an eight-month hiatus during which I was so sick. I am thinking, between bursts of inspiration, about how essential passion is and has been to me during my life. How I never thought anything was of any value unless pursued with passion. How passion takes courage. The French poet Charles Baudelaire spoke of "the banal canvas of our pitiful lives." Since I first read those words, I have always said to myself: "Throw some paint on your canvas! Some fuchsia! Some periwinkle!" I have realized, through the decades, to what extent passion requires commitment, and for writing in particular. The German poet Rainer Maria Rilke described this aspect of passion, in particular the passion to write, best. In his *Letters to a Young Poet*, Rilke advised the young poet Franz Kappus to "ask yourself in the most silent hour of your night: *must* I write? Dig into yourself for a deep answer. And . . . if you meet this solemn question with a strong, simple '*I must*,' then build your life in accordance with this necessity . . ."

I am looking at my computer screen at this very moment and reflecting on the importance of passions in life, about which I have just been writing. As I see it, passions have a life of their own, without context, existing as an end and not a means to one, depending on nothing for their existence but their very selves. Passions for passions' sake, if you like. They have always kept me going and engaged in life. And especially after getting a new heart, they mean more to me than ever.

A memory of a passion long buried surfaces. I have always loved the Swedish language, ever since I was first exposed to it as I watched one of Ingmar Bergman's subtitled films (*Wild*

Strawberries, I think) in my early teens. In my opinion, it is, with Portuguese, the most mellifluous of languages in which I am not fluent (not counting French and Italian, that is). Not to mention the fact that it is the native country of Björn Borg, Ingmar and Ingrid Bergman, August Strindberg, Emanuel Swedenborg, Alfred Nobel, Dag Hammarskjöld, Ingemar Stenmark, Annika Sörenstam, Ann-Margret, Anita Ekberg, Greta Garbo, Max von Sydow, Liv Ullmann, and Bibi Andersson. Since watching (and especially *hearing*) the Bergman film, I always had the passion to speak Swedish, but, sadly, neither the time nor the opportunity.

Until one evening in 1987, during an advertising class I was teaching at the School of Visual Arts, when I am noticing an attractive young student sitting at the back of the room. I am noticing her mostly because of her hair, which is thick, spiky, and flaming pinkish-purple (fuchsia? periwinkle?). After the class, we chat a bit—the first syllable that exits her mouth betrays the fact that she is Swedish—and she mentions that she can't afford to take the class and asks me if she could audit it. I agree to let her bend the rules, of course, but not before negotiating a quid pro quo, namely, that in return, she help me learn to speak Swedish.

Thereafter, we meet for breakfast in New York City once a week for three months, before I go to work. I purchase a book, *Essentials of Swedish Grammar*, which I study in whatever spare time I can carve out. Aside from being a helpful grammar guide, it offers me a host of phrases that most any earnest and conscientious tourist would find incredibly useful for basic communication needs. You know, phrases like *Jag känner att en myra kryper uppför mitt ben* ("I can feel that an ant is crawling up my leg") and

En liten elefant är större än en stor mygga ("A little elephant is bigger than a big mosquito"). But the pronunciation of many Swedish words can't be learned from a book, which is where my pinkish-purple-haired Swedish student-become-pedagogue comes in.

When our minicourse ends, I have a rudimentary grasp of Swedish, something I treasure, because it is the passion to speak the language that propelled and impelled me to learn it. In fact, thirteen years later (in 2000), I had the opportunity to live for two months in Solna, a suburb of Stockholm, during which (yay!) I was able to express myself, albeit bumblingly: *Hur är det? Hej då. Var är toaletten?* Most important, I had finally satisfied my burning passion to (sorta) speak Swedish.

As the months pass, my new-and-improved routine is not dull or repetitive in the least. To the contrary, it is a great pleasure to plan out my days, to give them some structure once again, to have (even modest) goals. Up at six, writing from six to nine, breakfast at nine, cardiac rehab at ten, writing from eleven to one, lunch, writing from two to four, watching MSNBC and relaxing before dinner, dinner at seven, private time and TV from eight to eleven, sleep at eleven. In addition to periodic beach walks and guitar sessions and tennis (after fifty-six years of playing seriously, it has now been about eight years since I last played, so it is a great joy to return to the game I adore).

I am realizing that a regular routine has replaced my life in the hospital in one particularly salubrious way, among many obvious others: it has given me structure and goals and deadlines and something to look forward to every day. As opposed to my days in the hospital, which I passed as if I were a dog. Now don't get me wrong, I adore dogs a whole lot, but, unlike us, they have no sense of time or of making plans or of setting goals. Which is what I felt like in the hospital. My dog days (of spring and summer) oozed by, identical and nameless. I didn't lose track of time; rather, I had zero sense of it. Tuesday? What's *that*? Seconds, minutes, hours, days, weeks, months? *Huh?* It was all one formless blob, one faceless continuum, one structureless black hole. But now, all this has been replaced—mercifully—by passion, direction, focus, and goals once again.

Susan and I also return to making plans for the future. Attending my—gulp!—fiftieth college reunion (at times, we sure didn't think we'd make it, but make it we did, in June of 2016, and it was one of the joyous highlights of my life). Returning someday to our beloved Italy to visit our friends Giuseppe and Maria and kids Francesco and Filippo, Mauro and Antonella and son Augusto, and Tania and Marco (at times, we sure didn't think we'd make it, but make it we did, in October of 2016, and it was one of the most wonderful trips we ever took). Enjoying all our kids and grandchildren again.

Constantly, I am asking myself: *Should I even be here? How did I make it through all this?* It is all a ridiculous dream, an absurd piece of science fiction.

And another thing, inexplicable and stretching the boundaries of sci-fi. Aside from the improvements in appetite, sleep, endurance, energy, and strength bequeathed to me by my new heart, there is the strange matter of my right calf muscle. In the late-'80s, when I was in my midforties, I was playing in a three-on-three basketball game with five twentysomethings. I thought I could keep up with them easily, but then again, I also thought that I could eventually acquire a taste for brussels sprouts. I ended up tearing my right Achilles tendon badly, and my foot and most of my leg were in a cast for six months. The result of this crural incarceration was an atrophied right calf muscle, which never regenerated its original bulk. Until now. Somehow, as a result of my heart surgery and/or the meds I was taking subsequent to it, my calf muscle grew, miraculously, and is now virtually as big as its left counterpart.

Logic, shlogic.

I am learning new eating habits. I have given up (albeit kicking and screaming) certain pleasures, chief among them sushi and fried eggs (possible bacteria) and steak (possible bacteria in the pink part of medium-rare, although—faithfully obedient to Michelle Kittleson's liberal permission—I plan to consume one every so often). I have learned to eat veggies, but I have to draw the line at lima beans, asparagus, and brussels sprouts. And I have made Ak-Mak crackers, muesli, granola, hummus, lentils, turkey bacon, Jarlsberg Lite cheese, egg salad, Boost, tomatoes, apples, oranges, cottage cheese, lamb chops on the grill (medium), baked potatoes, whole-wheat pasta, mahi-mahi, sole, chicken-and-veggie kabobs, green beans, broccoli, peppers (red, yellow, and orange), and spinach integral parts of my weekly intake.

All in all, life is good. Well, let me rephrase that.

In our kitchen, Susan and I have this big, black, rounded ceramic heart that is coated with some chalkboard material. (We purchased the heart years ago, well before my transplant experience, so it means so much more to us today.) Attached to it is a string, at the end of which a piece of white chalk is tied onto it. We have used this heart to write occasional messages to each other, some gooily sentimental, some newsworthy, most intended to be either witty or inspirational or just plain silly.

One day a few years ago, Susan wrote on the heart three simple and therapeutic words: "Life is good!" At some point as I passed by the heart, I must have brushed against it klutzily, smudging the final chalky letter of the uplifting phrase. So from then on, and especially now, we laugh about and treasure what remained of that message on the heart (the altered message remains to this day) to express our appreciation of being happy and healthy (and also, as a double-entendre bonus, of the fact that human existence is flawed and imperfect and, yes, often messy):

Life is goo!

I am well aware that I am living on borrowed time, as the saying goes. That every day is a miracle for me and that it is my *sacred duty* to enjoy every single one as much as I possibly can. I have discovered on Google that the survival rate in America for heart transplant patients is about 50 percent after ten years. This is the time period I'm most interested in, since I'll be eighty-one in 2025, which is now four years over the life expectancy of transplantless American males. A fifty-fifty chance of reaching that age! Well, I'll take those odds any day of the week. Life is, after all, a fifty-fifty affair, right? Survival is pretty much a crapshoot, especially as the years roll by. The glass is always half-full and half-empty. The odds for anything, including survival, pretty much even out, as do the good and the bad breaks. What goes around comes around. The two sides of the proverbial coin. Bla bla bla. So I am determined to make it *at least* to 2025. And since I am an eternal optimist and since I have promised Susan that I'd live to ninety, I am, deep in the recesses of my mind, already planning my gala 2034 birthday party!

One day, during a long walk with Susan on a Carlsbad beach a few months after my transplant surgery, I decide once and for all to move forward on something that Susan has been urging me to do: although I have been writing novels for the last dozen years, I will embark on an unfamiliar adventure and write a memoir centering around all that I have gone through the past many months. It was such a life-changing event, truly, that it is screaming out to be recorded. Yes, I will write all about it. I will share my inner thoughts with myself and with others. I will tell the story of how my coronary ordeal has made me think even more meaningfully about many of life's profound and universal paradoxes that have preoccupied my mind the past six decades or so: fear and hope, despair and joy, failure and success, pride and humility, control and surrender, arbitrariness and justice, constriction and freedom, youth and age, life and death. I will express my feelings about self-belief and optimism and passion and how I feel in my heart that they will always prevail in the face of challenges, hardships, even imminent death. I will hope it helps others who find themselves in a similar situation, and their families and friends and acquaintances and colleagues. I will hope it helps cardiologists and other physicians and medical professionals to be even more empathetic than they already are toward their patients. I will hope it is read and enjoyed by people who think deeply about life and all its conflicts and mysteries. I will title the book *Time for a Heart-to-Heart: Reflections on Life in the Face of Death*.

I will hope that someday it will get published . . .

13
Luggage Rack

My lips disappear as I squeeze them tight, exposing my top six front teeth. I scrunch up both cheeks until they hurt—just the way Bogie does whenever he has a belt onscreen. A sip of Balvenie (my first single malt in five months) slides down my throat, both shocking and soothing my system. I am wearing my favorite pair of Levi's and a light-and-dark-blue-striped "Italia 1982 campioni del mondo" ("Italy 1982 world champions") soccer T-shirt, sitting in our Swedish rocking chair, and gazing at reproductions of some of my favorite works of art on the walls of our modest living room in Carlsbad: a Picasso, a Rembrandt, three little Blakes, a Searle, two Tarkays, and four Susan Ellen Loves. I am listening to a CD of Handel's sonatas for flute and harpsichord. I am blissfully letting sink in everything that has happened to me during my entire ordeal and recovery—the Good, the Bad, and the Ugly. Mostly the Good. I am hearing in my head the voice of Lou Gehrig, as ALS was ravaging his body, in his famous Yankee Stadium farewell address of 1939: "Fans, for the past two weeks you have been reading about the bad break I got. Yet today I consider myself the luckiest man on the face of the earth."

Indeed.

I am beginning to put things in a brand-new perspective, as I get back in the swing of things and revisit the raw realities of life. Financial issues? Small potatoes! Side effects of my medications? Drops in the bucket! Annoying calls from telemarketers? Fuhgettaboutit!

I am savoring every little thing in my life now. I have had no rejections or infections or infarctions, my chest wounds are nearly healed and minimally painful, my biopsy and blood test numbers are looking good, my MRIs have revealed not a single cancer cell floating around inside of me, I am thinking more clearly, the food tastes better (my appetite is ridiculous), I am sleeping better, I have much more energy and stamina, I am appreciating the flora and fauna and sun and clouds and sky and ocean more than ever. And every big thing: my amazing wife, Susan; my incredible kids Noah, Jenny, and Sarah; my cherished grandchildren Stephen, Gavon, Lila, and Emmy; my loving son- and daughter-in-law Eric and Carol and stepdaughter and husband Elissa and Dan; my beloved close friends (you know who you are); and my passions for writing, reading, sports, music, art, literature, travel, food and wine, dogs . . .

I am appreciating all the lessons I have learned through my adventure, how they have deepened my understanding of everything I have endured in the past, what they have taught me about the greater meaning of my experience here on Earth and of the challenges, pain, and conflicts that life has a way of throwing at me, at all of us.

A second sip of my dark amber nectar, another glance at the Picasso etching, and a homespun yet deeply profound line from a George Strait song suddenly pops into my head: "I ain't never saw a hearse with a luggage rack."

One of the reasons I love country music is that, despite the (sometimes charming) questionable grammar and (sometimes charming) cloying sentimentality, it occasionally produces a lyric so oddball and hysterical and profound that, shoot, it could make you drive your car clear off the dadgum road when you listen to it. Which is precisely what nearly happened to me when I first heard Strait warble those lyrics.

George's words are now making me think about material things and how much less they mean to me now in the perspective and through the prism of my recent challenge, of my having clung to life in the face of death. Not to say I don't appreciate certain possessions—my Guild DV-72 and Martin 000-28EC guitars, for instance, and my books and my old tennis racquets and our little garden and our art and our CDs. But if every one of these things should suddenly disappear from the face of the planet, I would still feel like Lou Gehrig did when he gave that speech.

After all, as George Carlin would say, it's only *stuff*.

A third sip of my Balvenie. I am reflecting now on the wisdom of a quote from Thoreau: "Simplify, simplify." two gloriously—and simply!—redundant words that emphasize what little we humans really need to survive (on Walden Pond or in Carlsbad, CA, or wherever) and to enjoy life to the fullest.

In the same vein, I am pondering those well-worn verses from Omar Khayyám's Rubáiyát:

> *Here with a Loaf of Bread beneath the Bough,*
> *A Flask of Wine, a Book of Verse—and Thou*
> *Beside me singing in the Wilderness—*
> *And Wilderness is Paradise enow.*

The simple things in life should be enough for us all, shouldn't they? I know that seems "simplistic" and naive, because it is a concept that is in conflict with all of our lives, which are by definition complex and filled with distractions and obligations and, well, "sleeping policemen." But one thing I do know, if I know nothing else: after what I've been through, when put in perspective, life doesn't have to be all that complicated. It doesn't have to be brain surgery.

Or even heart surgery.

Afterword

The accounts of Bob Mitchell as he experienced heart attacks, irregular heartbeats with lifesaving shocks from his implantable defibrillator, and the threat of needing a mechanical device to support his failing heart illustrate the ordeal that patients with severe heart disease often undergo. This is even more sobering when you consider that these challenges are only the prelude to the arduous journey that is heart transplantation.

The wait for a donor heart is indeed agonizing, as one can only hope that a donor heart will come in time. Bob describes how he navigates through the long wait for a donor heart by deftly associating remembrances of events that shaped his life and helped him brave the unknown. In addition to his heart disease, Bob had a scare with kidney cancer, which fortunately was removed and did not compromise his candidacy for heart transplantation. Anyone else may have quit, but Bob persevered with positive thoughts to keep the possibility of a second chance alive.

As a transplant physician, I have had the privilege to witness the miracle of transplantation firsthand. It never ceases to amaze me what the human body can endure and the resiliency that the human mind can encompass to continue the drive to survive and in fact thrive. Bob's story is a testament to this. What touches me most about Bob's story is the support and love from his wife, Susan. Transplantation is not something that happens to one person—it happens to a whole family. Indeed, it is so difficult to go through all the suffering of a severe illness without someone to be there for you and to hold your hand. This relationship is literally a lifeline, and the story between Bob and Susan epitomizes this special force in the human spirit.

I believe that Bob's story will provide hope to other patients with severe medical diseases, promote faith in modern medicine, and, above all, underscore the importance of support from family and friends to healing and recovery. This book is about real life and a great and hard-fought outcome, as told by a true novelist. The dictionary tells us that the primary meaning of transplant is to "lift and reset in another situation." In a very real way, Bob has managed to lift and reset all of us in the telling of his story, and we are fortunate to find ourselves in a place of renewed gratitude and appreciation for having come along for the ride.

Dr. Jon A. Kobashigawa
Director of the Heart Transplant Program; Thomas D. Gordon
Professor of Medicine, Cedars-Sinai Medical Center, LA
February 2017

Acknowledgments

In the typical Acknowledgments section at the end of a book, the expressions "from the bottom of my heart," "my heartfelt thanks," and "this book wouldn't have been possible without the help of" are all well-meaning and sincere, but nonetheless hyperbolic and figurative in meaning.

In my case, regarding the first group of people to whom I owe an enormous amount of gratitude, these same words are meant to be literal in meaning and rooted firmly in reality. And so, from the bottom of my heart, my heartfelt thanks to the following physicians at the Cedars-Sinai Medical Center in LA, the talented, brilliant, and empathetic people who saved my life in so many ways and without whose help, advice, and support, quite literally, this book—not to mention the remaining chapters of my life—wouldn't have been possible: the amazing cardiology team (Jon Kobashigawa, Dael Geft, Michele Hamilton, Michelle Kittleson, Jignesh Patel, David Chang, Jaime Moriguchi, Mamoo Nakamura, Lawrence Czer, Babak Azarbal, and Antoine Hage) and my amazing surgeons (Irene Kim, kidney transplant; Hyung Kim, kidney cancer surgery and nephrectomy; and Alfredo Trento, heart transplant, ably assisted by Paul Perry and Paula Ruiz). Not to mention (but I will) nephrologist Larry Froch, pulmonologist Michael Levine, endocrinologist Conrad Tseng, and social worker Sara Morrison. As well as the caring and committed team of Nurse Coordinators and RNs. And, of course, my extraordinarily supportive cardiologist at Scripps La Jolla, Ajay Srivastava.

That was AD (Avoiding Death); this is BC (Before Cedars): my gratitude also to the cardiologists who have kept my heart beating literally, during the past thirty years, with their caring and their expertise—Stuart Seides, Avraham Merav, Michael Feld, George Smith, Alan Brown, and Michael Shehata.

A postoperative shout-out to the terrific cardiac rehabilitation team at Tri-City Wellness Center in Carlsbad, CA, who kept my spirits up and my heart racing again, during my four grueling but invigorating rehab months: Dr. Sharon Slowik, Jennifer Brown, Chris Cooperman, April Arcaris, Ricky Harm, Jill Willingham, and Janice Bachar.

Many thanks, from the heart, to the outstanding team at Skyhorse Publishing: to Publisher Tony Lyons, Group Editorial Director Mark Gompertz, and editor Mike Lewis, for initially believing in and supporting this book project; to my superb editor, Caroline Russomanno, for her considerable editorial skills and her shepherding prowess; to Madeleine Ball, my energetic publicist, for her competence and her industry; to Sarah Jones, author liaison, for her cheerful and efficient assistance; and to designer Rain Saukas, who so powerfully adapted the 1890 painting I submitted to him, *Anatomía del corazón* by Spanish artist Enrique Simonet y Lombardo, which proudly adorns the cover of this book.

Warm cardiac thank-yous to Larry King for his kind words in the foreword, to Dr. Jon A. Kobashigawa for his lovely afterword, and to Dr. Craig R. Smith, Dr. Stuart F. Seides, and Dr. Mike Roizen for their much-appreciated and generous blurbs.

A special expression of gratitude to my dear friends who have helped keep my heart beating figuratively, with their loyalty and their love: Hank and Elayne Gardstein, Lance and Mary Donaldson-Evans (and Andrew and Catherine), Frank and Barbara Fleizach, Ken and Paula Horn, Anthony Caprio, Bill and Beth Jaquith, Pete and Linda Haller, Stan and Carroll Possick, Meredith Geisler, Suzanne Nash, David and Joanne Frantz, Ann von Gal and Louie Neiheisel, Seymon and Lynne Ostilly, Bob Joseph and Val Light, Mike and Sandy Appelbaum, Chuck and Barbara Debevoise, Alan and Bonnie Gorfin, Alison Archer, Adriene Rudy Fern, Gil and Barbara Feldman, David Lee Rubin, Bob and Fran Rubin, Jim and Judy Kramer, Pete and Kris Allen, John and Jane Gould, Budge and Kyle Upton, Bob and Kathi Roesler, Alan Pearlman, Wink Willett, Marty Wasserman, Hal Crowther and Lee Smith, George and Marie Pistorius, Fred and Dottie Rudolph, Diane Cabaud (and Nicole and Simone), Joe and Bev Gerber, Robin Landa, Fred Thaler and Linda Kaplan, Nat and Ann Greenfield, Ernie and Amy Fleishman, Kip and Janet Pope, Peter Bregman, David and Gail Nathanson, Joel Drucker, Howard Rogg, David and Ellie deVries, Ray and Gini La Charité, Allan and Dallas Pasco, Russ and Kathy Doherty, Steve Weinstock, Jenny Lewis, Carol Turturro, Alan Zahn, Randy Hecht, John and Martha Storey, and Chuck Perrin.

A heartfelt cheers, *mille mercis, grazie mille,* and *toda raba* to my equally wonderful overseas friends, who have so often filled my heart with joy: Mark Cripps, Hugh Herbert-Burns, Frédéric and Judith Bluysen, Giuseppe Signorile and Maria Gravina (and Francesco and Filippo), Mauro Cazzaro and Antonella Maione (and Augusto), Marco Croci and Tania Calcinaro, Antonietta Cisterna, Marcello Olivari and Antonella Timpano, Umberto Cipriani and Angelica Fraulo, Leo and Margaret Schwartz (and Ruthie and Daniel), and Rony and Rachel Herz.

I am so grateful to my bighearted family for their love and support: Stan and Phyllis Clurman (and Mara and Bruce), Dan and Elissa Goodkin (and Lila and Emmy), Phil and Shelley London (and Adam and Jordan), and the Finkelstein cousins: Lee (and Evel), Ellen (and Doug), Eric (and Gail), and Steven (and Nancy).

And to my incredible children, who have never failed to keep me feeling young at heart: Noah (and Carol and Stephen and Gavon), Jenny (and Eric), and Sarah.

Finally, what (more) can I say about my loving, giving, passionate, ebullient, funny, creative, and talented wife, soul mate, and main heartthrob, Susan Ellen Love? Without you, sweetie, I am certain I would never have survived this cardiological ordeal (and, for that matter, life in general). You fill my heart with such love, joy, laughter, and peace that I am now, for the first time in a very long time, at a total and complete loss for words . . .

Again, from the bottom of my heart, a great big thank-you to all of the above, who, to paraphrase the immortal Yogi Berra, have made this book necessary.

About the Author

Bob Mitchell's memoir *Time for a Heart-to-Heart* is a reflection of his remarkably eclectic life experience. He has been a sports fanatic since birth and is also passionate about writing, reading, art, music, world literature, travel, food and wine, and dogs. He is the author of eleven published books, including four volumes of literary criticism, a collection of poems, a volume of essays, a collection of prose poems, and three novels about sports and the meaning of life. Bob studied at Williams (BA), Columbia (MA), and Harvard, where he earned a PhD in French and Comparative Literature. Fluent in four languages, he taught in France for a year on a Fulbright Fellowship and has had careers as a university French professor (Harvard, Purdue, Ohio State), a teaching tennis pro, an award-winning advertising creative director, a teacher of advertising and creative writing (New York, Paris, Tel Aviv, Jerusalem), and a novelist. Bob has lived in seven states as well as Paris, Brittany, Angers, Besançon, London, Florence, Stockholm, Montreal, and Tel Aviv and currently resides in Carlsbad, CA, with his wife, artist Susan Ellen Love.